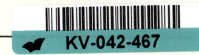

TREATMENT OF THE JUVENILE SEX OFFENDER

NEUROLOGICAL AND PSYCHIATRIC IMPAIRMENTS

Matthew L. Ferrara, Ph.D.
and
Sherry McDonald, L.M.S.W.-A.C.P.

JASON ARONSON INC.
Northvale, New Jersey
London

Production Editor: Ruth E. Brody

This book was set in 11-point English Times by TechType of Upper Saddle River, New Jersey, and printed and bound by Book-mart Press of North Bergen, New Jersey.

Library of Congress Cataloging-in-Publication Data

Ferrara, Matthew L.
    Treatment of the juvenile sex offender: neurological and psychiatric impairments / by Matthew L. Ferrara and Sherry McDonald.
        p. cm.
    Includes bibliographical references and index.
    ISBN 1-56821-566-5 (alk. paper)
    1. Teenage sex offenders — Rehabilitation. 2. Adolescent psychotherapy — Residential treatment. 3. Learning disabled teenagers — Rehabilitation. I. McDonald, Sherry. II. Title.
    [DNLM: 1. Juvenile Delinquency — psychology. 2. Residential Treatment — in adolescence. 3. Sex Offenses — psychology. 4. Nervous System Diseases — in adolescence. 5. Mental Disorders — in adolescence.   WS 463 F374t 1995]
    RJ506.S48F47   1995
    616.85'83 — dc20
    DNLM/DLC   95-14354

Manufactured in the United States of America. Jason Aronson Inc. offers books and cassettes. For information and catalog write to Jason Aronson Inc., 230 Livingston Street, Northvale, New Jersey 07647.

DATE DUE

Demco, Inc. 38-293

TREATMENT OF THE JUVENILE SEX OFFENDER

CONTENTS

INTRODUCTION

One of the most beleaguered and embattled arenas in contemporary health care is the psychiatric residential treatment center. While the entire health care industry seems to be under scrutiny and in a state of flux, residential treatment centers are suffering a particularly devastating assault. In most residential treatment centers, layoffs are so common that business euphemisms such as "downsizing" or "rightsizing" are commonplace. Professionals in these settings find themselves stretched as they take on administrative tasks or begin cross-training so that they can work in more than one of the programs at their facility where staff shortages exist due to "rightsizing." All of these struggles might go unnoticed by the sex offender therapist if it were not for the ever-increasing scope of treatment for juvenile sex offenders.

The field of sex offender treatment is a burgeoning field. Perhaps this is the result of the rapid growth in the corrections industry. There can be no doubt that correctional budgets are increasing with each passing year and this trend does not show any signs of weakening. As a result, correctional programs enjoy the availability of funding. In particular, sex offender treatment services have benefited from the growth in the correctional industry. A recent survey identified 755 specialized treatment programs for juvenile sex offenders in the United States alone (Knopp et al. 1992). All this suggests that treatment for juvenile sex offenders is well established and well funded, at least as compared to services and programs in the health care industry. Unfortunately, this is beginning to become more problematic.

Due to the proliferation of sex offender treatment, the trend is for programs to become increasingly specialized. Consider the role that the residential treatment center might play in this scenario. The residential treatment center could fill the niche of treating the neurologically or psychiatrically impaired juvenile sex offender. The specialized services and professional staff routinely found at a residential treatment center are ideally suited for treating this clientele. Yet the layoffs and decreased funding that threaten the operations of these facilities undermine the potential for successful treatment. Despite the obstacles that exist, the residential treatment center still remains the placement of choice for the neurologically and psychiatrically impaired juvenile sex offender.

The treatment program described in this book is one of but a few juvenile sex offender programs for the neurologically and psychiatrically impaired. The program was conceptualized and developed in the turbulent vortex of health care reform, reduced insurance coverage, and shrinking budgets. An equilibrium had to be achieved between the pressures caused by changes in the industry and the demand to provide effective treatment to a high-risk population. Although the program continues to evolve, the existing program as described in this book has achieved an equilibrium, and hopefully, in doing so, it may have established a blueprint whereby other programs may be developed.

The first chapter in this book delineates the population served by the program. The neurologically and psychiatrically impaired juvenile sex offender is identified as the target population for the program. Since little research has been aimed at this population, the existing literature was scrutinized in an effort to adduce relevant information about the neurological functioning of juvenile sex offenders.

Because so little research has been conducted regarding the neurological functioning of juvenile delinquents, the treatment program described in this book could not be based exclusively on empirical findings. Rather, the program had to be conceptually driven. Chapter 2 contains an etiological theory for deviant sexual behavior. Although the program described in this book focuses on the juvenile sex offender with neurological and psychiatric impairments, the etiological theory described in this chapter pertains to all types of sex offenders: adolescent, adult, neurologically intact, high risk, and others. Much of the existing literature regarding sexual behavior and sexual deviance is discussed in the context of this theory. Fields as diverse as sociobiology and endocrinology are discussed along with the more familiar topics of thinking errors and disinhibitors.

In Chapter 3, techniques for working with the neurologically impaired juvenile sex offenders are discussed. The chapter opens with the presentation of a general strategy for working with this clientele. It is suggested that much of what is known of the psychodynamic description of the primitive personality may apply to the neurologically impaired client. After discussing the commonalities between treating the neurologically impaired client and the primitive personality, guidelines are presented for intervening with the neurologically impaired juvenile. Frequently encountered neurological deficits are identified. Techniques to circumvent the disabling effects of these impairment are presented. The special techniques discussed in this chapter are likened to bridges that span the gaps in the client's ability to function. Hence, the program based upon these techniques has been dubbed the *Bridges Program*.

Chapter 4 integrates all the information presented in the preceding chapters. In this chapter, a program narrative is offered that describes the treatment program for juvenile sex offenders with neurological impairments. Included is a discussion of the therapeutic tasks that compose the treatment program. Detailed information is offered regarding therapeutic tasks, and the ultimate goal is to enable the clinician to work effectively within the guidelines as described in this chapter.

Chapter 5 describes a sex offender treatment program for

juvenile sex offenders without neurological impairments. It is assumed that a residential treatment center may wish to specialize and offer a program for neurologically impaired offenders; however, most residential treatments have a diverse clientele. Due to the diversity of the clients at a facility, it could be expected that a sizable percentage would not have neurological impairments. Hence, these clients without neurological impairments could benefit from more traditional sex offender treatment. Chapter 5 is a program narrative of a juvenile sex offender treatment program for youths who are not neurologically impaired. This program is designed for use with typical juvenile sex offenders and juvenile sex offenders with mild psychiatric conditions, such as dysthymia, attention deficit disorder, or post-traumatic stress disorder. The program described in this chapter is very similar to the Bridges Program. Therefore, persons trained in one program could readily work in the other. Since professionals who work in residential treatment centers are often asked to work in more than one of the facility's programs, the similarities between these two programs will be welcomed.

Chapter 6 discusses milieu management. Specifically, some of the more common manipulative ploys that juvenile sex offenders utilize are discussed. Guidelines are offered for preventing and responding to these ploys.

We wanted this book to have a decidedly applied emphasis. For this reason, we included an appendix that contains the client workbook for the two sex offender programs described in the book. Each client workbook is a compendium of therapeutic tasks that a client must complete to graduate from the program. This appendix should be welcomed by those readers who put a premium on books that emphasize a practical "how to" approach.

In closing, we would like to extend our support to those who would endeavor to implement the program described in this book. Developing and implementing this program was quite taxing for the authors. If it were not for the vision and support offered by the administrators at the San Marcos Treatment Center and the parent company, Healthcare America, this program would never have been developed. We only hope that readers receive as much support should they embark on a similar effort.

Matthew L. Ferrara, Ph.D.
Sherry McDonald, L.M.S.W.-A.C.P.

1

Scope of the Problem

A voluminous body of literature exists regarding the juvenile sex offender. Much is known about these offenders, their victims, and the nature of their behavior. Treatment programs have proliferated, and consequently the factors associated with successful rehabilitation of juvenile sex offenders have begun to emerge. The treatment programs currently being developed are beginning to specialize, and specific treatment programs exist for juvenile sex offenders with mental retardation, substance abuse problems, and violent acting out. Despite the increasing literature and the proliferation of treatment programs, the juvenile sex offender with neurological or psychiatric impairments has received little attention.

Juvenile sex offenders with psychiatric or neurological impairments do exist (Tarter et al. 1983). A surprisingly small number of researchers and clinicians use these variables as a means for identifying subgroups among juvenile sex offenders. Failure to identify subgroups based on these variables has undoubtedly skewed the results of many research projects and undermined the integrity of many treatment programs. Despite the necessity to recognize and respond to neurological and psychiatric impairments, there is little to suggest that clinicians or researchers attend to this variable.

A review of the literature pertaining to the neurological and psychiatric functioning of juvenile sex offenders is presented here. The issue of neurological impairments will be addressed first; then psychiatric functioning will be discussed. As there is little in the literature that directly addresses the neurological functioning of juvenile sex offenders, literature that provides indirect information is included in the review. A chronological approach is taken in which the early literature is reviewed first and then a discussion of the contemporary literature is offered.

NEUROLOGICAL FUNCTIONING

There were no computed tomography (CT) scans, positron emission tomography (PET) scans, or magnetic resonance imaging (MRI) in 1950. Not surprisingly, there are no studies of juvenile sex offenders that reveal brain functioning or map topographical regions of the brain. Even with the expectation that sophisticated methodologies would not be used during this time period, the research pertaining to the neurological functioning of juvenile sex offenders is surprisingly sparse. In fact, in the 1950s and 1960s there were no research efforts that focused exclusively upon the neurological functioning of juvenile sex offenders. During this era there is, however, some research that pertains to the intellectual and academic functioning of juvenile sex offenders. Since this literature can provide indirect evidence of neurological functioning, a few of the more noteworthy studies are discussed. The purpose of this discussion is to demonstrate that even the early research provides indirect evidence of neurological impairment of juvenile sex offenders.

Markey (1950) studied twenty-five boys and twenty-five girls referred to a juvenile court for sexual misconduct that endangered the "morals of the culprit, the victim or the community" (p. 719) The methodology of this study entailed a psychiatric interview and use of the Rorschach. When compared with other same-aged delinquents who did not engage in sexual misconduct, the juvenile sex offender was found to be of similar age and IQ. The finding pertaining to IQ scores is of interest because IQ scores and neurological functioning are related. That is, neurological impairments result in poor performance on IQ tests. Based upon this study there is no apparent indirect evidence of neurological problems among juvenile sex offenders.

Atcheson and Williams (1954) reviewed the records of 112 juvenile delinquents referred to a Canadian court between 1936 and 1948. Using the Stanford-Binet IQ test, male sex offenders were compared with non-sex offender delinquents. The juvenile sex offenders were found to have an average IQ score of 91.9 as compared with 94.5 for the non-sex offending males. In addition to having slightly lower IQ scores, the sex offenders were also found to have more variability in IQ subtests, standard deviation of 17.7 and 14.9, respectively. Furthermore, 25.2 percent of male sex offenders had IQ scores below 80 as compared with 11.1 percent among the control group. Based upon these findings, it would appear that there is some indirect evidence of cognitive impairment among juvenile delinquents. In particular, juvenile sex offenders appear to have lower scores than other delinquents. The variability of these IQ scores suggests that there may be several subgroups of juvenile sex offenders, for example, neurologically impaired and neurologically intact.

The two foregoing studies are fairly characteristic of the research that was conducted in the 1950s. Archival research, or review of existing records, was the most common means of collecting data. When test instruments were used, the Rorschach and Stanford-Binet tests were typically employed. Sophisticated measures of neuroanatomy and neurophysiology were not available. In fact, the Wechsler scales of intelligence were just being developed in the 1950s and these scales were not used extensively.

The research in the 1960s did not differ significantly from that in the 1950s. When the issue of juvenile sex offenders was put under scientific scrutiny, archival research, case studies, and an occasional standardized psychological test served as the methodology. For example, Maclay (1960) reviewed the files of twenty-nine boys who were referred to a juvenile court for sexual misconduct. The author did not interview or test the subjects in this study. He merely reviewed their files and reported some anecdotal information. Maclay concluded that male juvenile sex offenders come from homes with poor emotional support and the offenders themselves tend to be insecure. However, Maclay found reason for optimism as "in the great majority the boy's subsequent sexual development appears to have been good" (p. 190).

A more rigorous study of offender and offense characteristics was conducted later in the 1960s (Shoor et al. 1966). Like the other studies being conducted at this time, the study employed the method of archival review. The unique aspect of this study was that the authors did not rely exclusively on archival data. They also used interviews to collect data. The authors interviewed a variety of people including the perpetrator, his parents, his probation officer, and others having knowledge of the case. These authors discovered that the educational achievement of juvenile sex offenders tended to be low to fair. The authors noted that the juvenile sex offenders' academic performance was always below capacity.

As was the case in the 1950s, researchers in the 1960s also failed to conduct studies that directly examined the neurological functioning of juvenile sex offenders. Some of the studies during this time did examine IQ scores and academic functioning. These studies found results similar to those produced in the 1950s. That is, juvenile sex offenders performed below average on standard tests of intellectual functioning. This finding cannot be dismissed as resulting from situational factors. The research during this time demonstrated that the subaverage performance of delinquents on standardized measures of intelligence could not be explained solely in terms of race (Wolfgang et al. 1972) or social class

(Moffit et al. 1981). When external factors are eliminated, then the delinquent's poor performance on IQ tests must be explained in terms of intrapersonal factors, and neurological impairment may be the single best explanatory variable.

The 1970s brought with them the first study that used neurological factors as a variable (Lewis et al. 1979). In this study, sexually assaultive juvenile males were compared with violent non-sexually assaultive males. The authors used a variety of standardized psychological tests including the Wechsler Intelligence Scale for Children (WISC), Bender-Gestalt, Woodcock Reading Mastery Tests, and Key Math Diagnostic Arithmetic Test. Whenever possible, a sleep EEG was performed. The results revealed that 23.5 percent of the sexual assaulters and 3.3 percent of the violent offenders had grossly abnormal EEGs or grand mal seizures. These two groups did not differ on Full Scale, Verbal, or Performance IQ scores. Sexual assaulters performed less well on the reading test as compared with violent offenders, 5.59 and 3.95 years below grade level, respectively. Overall, both types of offenders exhibited neurological abnormalities and the authors concluded that violence of any kind and sexual violence per se may reflect similar underlying neurological vulnerabilities.

This study is important in that it is among the first studies to examine neurological impairment among juvenile sex offenders. The results of this study should have been anything but surprising to the authors as previous research did reveal that juvenile delinquents in general (Krgnicki 1978, Pontius and Ruttiger 1976, Stevens et al. 1968), and violent juvenile offenders in particular (Spellacy 1977) exhibit neurological impairments. What is surprising is that a subset of juvenile sex offenders could be identified as neurologically impaired and that this spurred little, if any, future investigation of this issue in the years to come. This is unfortunate as there was a theory of delinquency that posited delinquency was the result of a developmental lag in frontal lobe development. Pontius (1974) hypothesized that immature frontal lobe development could be detected using the EEG. The combination of the Pontius theory and the work of Lewis and colleagues (1979) might have resulted in some fruitful discoveries. This did not, however, occur.

The research conducted in the past fifteen years does not bring with it a dramatic increase in the number of studies that use sophisticated measures of neurological functioning of juvenile sex offenders. In some ways the contemporary research regarding juvenile sex offenders is reminiscent of the early research, especially with regard to the limited attention researchers give to neurological factors. The lack of attention given to neurological factors associated with juvenile sex offenders stands in stark contrast to the neurological research of juvenile delinquency in general. This research is sophisticated and detail oriented, whereas neurological research of juvenile sex offenders is almost nonexistent.

Given the paucity of studies that directly assess the neurological functioning of juvenile sex offenders, one is left with the task of finding indirect support for the nature and extent of neurological impairments among juvenile sex offenders. Two variables commonly discussed in the literature that provide indirect evidence of neurological functioning are cognitive functioning and psychiatric conditions.

COGNITIVE FUNCTIONING

An individual's performance test of intelligence is determined by a number of factors including global intelligence, cognitive skills, and school experience. The first two of these factors are of particular interest because global intelligence and cognitive skills develop optimally when the individual does not have neurological problems. The presence of a neurological condition may inhibit cognitive development, and consequently IQ scores would be expected to be low, if not below average.

Although intelligence is not by itself a strong predictor of delinquency (Famularo et al. 1992), it is well known that delinquents tend to score low on standardized tests of intelligence. Some studies suggest that up to one third of all delinquents could be expected to have intellectual functioning that falls in the range of mild mental retardation (Schuster and Guggenheim 1982). One rather consistent finding in the literature pertaining to juvenile delinquents is that performance IQ scores tend to be greater than verbal IQ scores. In terms of neurological functioning, this suggests that juvenile delinquents may have left-hemispheric disturbances.

Whereas the literature pertaining to IQ scores and delinquency is fairly well articulated, only a few studies have examined the intellectual functioning of juvenile sex offenders. Tarter and colleagues (1983) compared juvenile sex offenders to juvenile delinquents. No differences on a standardized test of intelligence was found. Saunders and colleagues (1986) discovered that violent juvenile sex offenders tended to have lower IQ scores than nonviolent juvenile sex offenders. The association of low IQ scores with violent behavior has been found with delinquents in general (Krgnicki 1978). When such a pattern has been discovered in the past, it is usually attributed to a higher incidence of neurological impairments among violent perpetrators (Kandel and Freed 1989).

Academic functioning is not exclusively determined by intellectual functioning or neurological functioning. There are a great many factors that affect academic achievement including truancy, parental support, and parental level of education. Still, there is one determinant of academic achievement that seems to have a neurological basis, that is, learning disorders. It is common knowledge that learning disabilities and below-average academic achievement are associated with neurological conditions. Dyslexia, dysgraphia, and other learning disabilities are known to have their neurological correlates. In some instances, the locus of neurological impairment is known for some learning disabilities.

In a study of 170 male adolescent sex offenders admitted to a residential treatment, over half of the offenders were below average in school performance (O'Brien 1988). Only 8 percent of the offenders admitted to the program had grade-appropriate academic performance. Sixty percent of the offenders were behind on their expected academic progress. Surprisingly, 32 percent of the offenders were above average. When the prevalence of learning disabilities among types of offenders was assessed, there were no differences among incest perpetrators, child molesters, and non–child sexual offenders, that is, 37 percent, 37 percent, and 38 percent, respectively. Overall, this study found that juvenile sex offenders do exhibit subaverage academic performance, but academic performance cannot be used as a variable to discriminate different types of offenders.

Other studies have also found that juvenile sex offenders lag behind in academic performance. Yet the prevalence of subaverage academic performance is not always as dramatic as that reported by O'Brien (1988). For example, Fehrenbach and colleagues (1986) examined 305 adolescent sex offenders and found only 32 percent to be lagging behind in academic achievement. In this sample 55 percent were on schedule and 2 percent were ahead of schedule.

As can be seen from a comparison of the O'Brien (1988) and Fehrenbach and colleagues (1986) studies, there is some disagreement regarding the exact prevalence of juvenile sex offenders who exhibit below-average academic performance. However, one finding is consistent across these studies: some juvenile sex offenders do exhibit below-average academic achievement. Those who work with juvenile delinquents will not view these findings as surprising. It is widely known that as a group, juvenile delinquents do poorly in school and frequently exhibit below-average academic performance. In a

study comparing juvenile sex offenders to juvenile delinquents who did not engage in sexual misconduct, no differences were found in reading, math, and spelling achievement
(Tarter et al. 1983).

Based upon the available literature, it appears that some
juvenile sex offenders do exhibit below-average academic
achievement. Perhaps more important is the finding that, on
average, 38 percent of these youthful offenders may be
diagnosed as learning disabled. Since learning disabilities and
poor academic achievement are both associated with neurological impairment, these findings indicate that some juvenile
sex offenders do suffer from neurological problems.

Performance on IQ tests and academic functioning do
provide indirect support for the contention that some juvenile sex offenders have neurological impairments. Still, it
should be recognized that these findings suggest a global or
generalized impairment. Research has yet to be conducted
with juvenile sex offenders that delineates specific types of
neurological impairments. There are, however, some studies
on non–sex offending juvenile delinquents that identify
specific types of neurological impairments.

Studies of the cognitive skills of non–sex offending juvenile delinquents have revealed two areas of deficit. Each area
of deficit may be related to impairments in different parts of
the brain. First, considerable literature exists that indicates
that delinquents have difficulties with certain executive functions including planning, abstraction, inhibition of inappropriate impulses, and cognitive flexibility (Moffit and Silva
1988, Yeudall et al. 1982). All of these difficulties have been
attributed to frontal lobe dysfunction. Second, juvenile
delinquents have exhibited difficulties with sequencing,
rhythmic functions, and expressive speech (Brinkman et al.
1984). These impairments have been attributed to brain
abnormalities in the temporal lobe region. Overall, it could
be expected that some juvenile sex offenders will have the
same neurological deficits known to exist in some juvenile

delinquents. If this proves to be true, then the research will likely discover at least two subtypes of neurologically impaired juvenile sex offenders: those with frontal lobe dysfunction and those with temporal lobe dysfunction.

PSYCHIATRIC CONDITIONS

One area of the juvenile sex offender literature that is quite rich is the description of offender characteristics. This literature provides information about offender functioning in a variety of areas including family relations, peer relations, interpersonal skills, and psychiatric functioning. Most of the literature regarding psychiatric functioning suggests that juvenile sex offenders have few psychological problems. A review of this literature is offered here.

Lewis and colleagues (1981) compared juvenile sex offenders with assaultive juvenile delinquents. They found no differences between these groups with regard to the presence of psychosis and depression. They did, however, find that on average, both groups of offenders exhibited high levels of emotional disturbance. The authors did not tie their observation of emotional disturbance to specific diagnostic categories.

Saunders and colleagues (1986) compared hands-off offenders (e.g., voyeurs) with child molesters and rapists. These authors did not use formal diagnostic labels but they did find some differences among offenders. Specifically it was discovered that hands-off offenders were deemed to be less disturbed than hands-on offenders. No comparison group was used.

In one study, a clinical examination of nineteen juvenile sex offenders was conducted (Becker et al. 1986). It was discovered that none of the offenders had even been hospitalized for a psychiatric problem, nor had anyone in their immediate families. Of the nineteen subjects interviewed, five had no *DSM-III* disorder, twelve were diagnosed with a conduct disorder, five with attention deficit disorder, four with a substance use disorder, two with an adjustment disorder, one with a dysthymic disorder, and one with a posttraumatic stress disorder. Even though some offenders had multiple diagnoses, it is noteworthy that no offenders were diagnosed with a thought disorder or a major affective disorder. The disorder that seems most closely related to neurological problems is the attention deficit disorder. This disorder was found in approximately 25 percent of the offenders.

Becker and colleagues' (1986) finding of no personal or family history of psychiatric treatment was replicated by Cavanagh Johnson (1988), who examined offenders as young as 4 years old. She concluded that child perpetrators exhibited little evidence of major psychopathology and no history of family psychiatric hospitalizations.

Bagley and Schewchuk-Dunn (1991) studied sixty individuals, ages 9 to 17, in two residential treatment centers for severely disturbed youths. These authors discovered that juvenile sex offenders, as compared to other children in the treatment centers, exhibited more hyperactivity, depression, and impulse disorder behaviors. These authors also claim that juvenile sex offenders exhibit more neurological problems than their non–sex offender counterparts. Specifically, 24 percent of the sex offenders as compared with 10 percent of the control group had a history of neurological problems such as seizure disorders.

Overall, it would appear that few juvenile sex offenders warrant a psychiatric diagnosis. A similar finding is evident in the literature regarding adult offenders (Murphy et al. 1992). For the most part, it would appear that youths do not engage in deviant sexual behavior as a result of psychiatric problems. Still, it is interesting to note the Bagley and Schewchuk-Dunn study, which reveals that when a juvenile sex offender is sufficiently disturbed to be placed in a residential treatment facility, he often appears more disturbed, hyperactive, and neurologically impaired than other youths at the facility. It may be that juvenile sex offenders who do warrant residential treatment are in fact severely disturbed. It is important to remember that none of the available research links juvenile sex offending with schizophrenia, severe depression, or other forms of major mental illness.

CONCLUSIONS

The literature regarding juvenile sex offenders spans half a century. Some aspects of the literature seem richly developed. For example, much is known about offenders' demographics, victim characteristics, and offense behaviors. Yet there are aspects of the research pertaining to juvenile sex offenders in which the issue is not one of finding "more" or "richer" information. Rather, the issue is one of finding some information. This is the situation with the literature pertaining to the neurological functioning of juvenile sex offenders.

It must be recognized that few studies exist that entail direct neurological measures of juvenile sex offenders. At best, one is left to act like a scientific sleuth finding clues and evidence regarding the neurological functioning of juvenile sex offenders. While indirect evidence does exist, the findings are meager and the data so inadequate that it is not yet possible to talk about specific areas of the brain that might promote sexual misconduct among youthful offenders. Such data are available for adults, although there are problems with this research as well. Still, one cannot help but be impressed by the scant information regarding the neurological functioning of juvenile sex offenders.

If anything can be gleaned from the literature, it is that a small percentage of juvenile sex offenders have neurological impairments. Based upon the research pertaining to IQ scores, academic achievement, and psychiatric conditions, it would appear that no more than 38 percent and perhaps closer to 25 percent of all juvenile sex offenders have some form of neurological impairment. The literature also suggests that if a juvenile sex offender has mental health problems that warrant placement in a residential treatment center, he is likely to look more dysfunctional and have a more disrupted past when compared with his non-sex offending peers in the treatment center (Bagley and Schewchuk-Dunn 1991).

The implications of these findings suggest that juvenile sex offenders with neurological impairments will continue to be unnoticed by researchers and clinicians. Furthermore, it is likely that the neurologically impaired juvenile sex offender who goes undetected will not attain the optional benefit from treatment due to problems in concentration, comprehension, and memory. Finally, it seems obvious that if a program is modified such that it can treat the neurologically impaired juvenile sex offender, program staff can expect to deal with clients who may appear more aggressive and more disturbed than other clients.

2

Etiological Considerations

The cause of sexual deviance is a much-debated topic. Despite all the interest and effort, a definitive explanation has yet to be attained. At best, the field can be characterized by competing hypotheses, some of which appear to account for a goodly portion of what is known about sexual deviance, while others fall far short of rendering a meaningful integration of the current knowledge.

As often happens, when an old puzzle is viewed from a different perspective, new solutions appear. In this book, the focus is upon the neurologically impaired person who engages in sexually deviant behavior. Looking at the etiological puzzle from the neuropsychological perspective has suggested a novel way of understanding the etiology of sexual deviance. It should be noted that although consideration of this issue began from the perspective of neuropathology, the resulting theory of sexual deviance applies to all forms and manifestations of sexual deviance, by all types of individuals: adolescents, adults, high IQ, mentally retarded, neurologically impaired, and neurologically intact.

At its most general level, the proposed theory of sexual deviance is quite simple and straightforward. It is assumed that two primary factors account for the occurrence of sexually deviant behavior: biological variables and socialization. Even though these two factors are identified separately in the theory, it is recognized that there is a reciprocal relationship between the biological variables and socialization: biological factors influence socialization and socialization influences biological factors. Many readers may be familiar with this dichotomy of variables and recognize it as the nature–nurture issue. A question that often arises when discussing the nature–nurture issue is: How much sexual deviance is due to biological factors and how much is due to socialization? Attempting to answer this question would probably be unproductive, if not impossible. The issue is not how much sexual deviance is apportioned to biological or socialization factors. Rather, the issue is how do these factors relate and affect each other as they shape human sexual behavior. Attempting to explain this issue is the goal of this chapter.

The etiological theory of sexual deviance assumes that sexual deviance, like all sexual behavior, begins with the sex drive (Figure 2–1). The sex drive is biologically based. It is the result of three very different influences: evolution, hormones, and neurological factors. These three factors are like

Figure 2.1

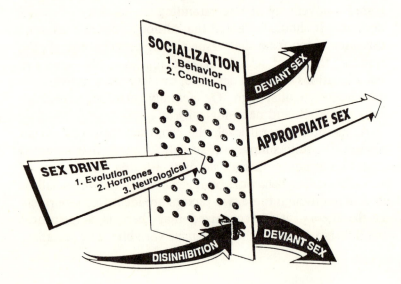

three strands that are wrapped together to form one rope. The separate strands each exert an independent influence; however, the influence of each of these strands is blended together such that a person experiences a single sex drive. Continuing with the analogy of the rope, when you pull on the rope, all strands of the rope pull together. In essence, all that you are aware of is the rope. Still, the rope is composed of separate strands. The sex drive is like the rope. It is difficult to tease apart the influence of each of these three factors, but that is precisely what is endeavored later in this chapter.

The second major factor in the theory of sexual deviance is socialization. All sexual values and sexual attitudes are learned and most sexual behavior is learned. Learning occurs naturally as an individual matures and becomes socialized. As a result of socialization, the individual acquires a set of standards that control the manner in which the biological sex drive is manifested. While socialization may vary from culture to culture, one thing remains constant: all societies impose standards for sexual behavior, and when one does not conform to these standards the individual is a deviate, or more precisely a sexual deviate. Socialization is learning and what is learned is a set of standards that inhibit the sex drive.

To really appreciate the effect of socialization, imagine that socialization is like a strainer that is used in a kitchen to wash vegetables. The water runs over the vegetables and out through the holes in the strainer. If the strainer is intact, no vegetables fall through. Socialization of sexual behavior is similar. The sex drive exerts pressure on the person to behave, but socialization acts like a strainer to ensure that only socially appropriate sexual behavior is manifested.

An important factor related to learning is disinhibition. Disinhibition clarifies how sexually deviant behavior can be exhibited by persons who have been fully socialized and possess the ability to engage in socially acceptable sexual behavior. Disinhibition can be thought of as a temporary neutralization of learning. Returning to the metaphor of the kitchen strainer, disinhibition can be thought of as a hole in the strainer through which more than just water escapes. Fortunately, the hole in the strainer, or disinhibition, is temporary and the learning can return to a fully integrated state capable of controlling the manner in which the sex drive is manifest.

The foregoing presentation describes the etiological theory of sexual deviance in broad brushstrokes. This general theory provides the structure into which much of what is known about sexual deviance can be integrated. The remainder of this chapter fills in the details of this theory by integrating information about human sexuality and sexual deviance. The discussion begins with the biological factors—evolution, hormones, and neurological factors. Then the issue of socialization is addressed. The chapter concludes with a discussion of the practical implications of this theory.

BIOLOGICAL FACTORS

It is important to understand that all sexual behavior, deviant as well as acceptable, begins with the biological sex drive. In this section, aspects of the sex drive as they pertain to sexual deviance are discussed. Each of the three components of the sex drive will be defined. The contemporary research and scientific theory about each factor will be discussed. Then the relationship of each factor to sexual deviance will be explored. This section demonstrates how evolution, hormones, and neurological factors support and promote deviant sexual behavior.

Evolution

The theory of evolution has not changed much since 1858 when Charles Darwin proposed that evolution occurs from a process called natural selection. Darwin used the term *natural selection* to contrast it with the term *artificial selection,* which referred to the reproduction of domestic animals that was controlled by humans. In natural selection, the forces of nature select who reproduces.

Many people know of Darwin's theory of evolution as "survival of the fittest." This phrase tends to create pictures of strong, dominating individuals reproducing while the weak languish without offspring. This is not entirely true. Contemporary biologists define fitness as reproductive success (Daly and Wilson 1983). Fitness does not refer to strength, speed, agility, or any other physical attribute. Fitness is simply the likelihood that an organism will survive to reproduce. Real fitness actually comes down to reproductive strategies: the individual with the most effective reproductive strategy produces the most offspring.

Reproductive strategy varies from species to species but all species, and all individuals, develop their reproductive strategy based upon two factors: mating effort and parenting effort. Mating effort refers to the effort exerted in finding, courting, and mating with a sexual partner. Parental effort refers to the amount of time and energy devoted to gestation, incubation, feeding, protecting, and teaching offspring. Some species expend little parental effort, for example, sharks. Humans appear to require the most parental effort to successfully enact their reproductive strategy.

While it may be obvious that different species have different reproductive strategies, different genders within a species may also have different reproductive strategies. The rule of thumb is that the gender that invests more parental effort will be selective about mating, whereas the gender that exerts minimal parental effort will breed indiscriminately. For example, Bateman (1948) showed that the male fruit fly increases reproductive success with multiple matings but the female does not. Bateman concluded that the male fruit fly relies on frequency of mating for reproductive success. Since

Bateman's early work, other sociobiologists studying other species have replicated his findings: repeated matings hold a reproductive advantage for males but not for females. Where fertilization and gestation occur inside the female, the female tends to be more discriminating than males in selecting mates. The pregnant female will have a tremendous investment in parental effort. Therefore, the female must carefully select mates to ensure that she avails herself of the best available gene pool.

If females are cautious in selecting mates, how do males select mates? Selection tends to occur on characteristics that suggest fertility. Some characteristics that might suggest fertility include youth, appealing appearance, and physical fitness. The male reproductive strategy is quite simple: reproduce with as many mates as possible, making sure that the mate appears fertile. Thus, male and female reproductive strategies are in conflict. The dilemma is how to resolve the conflict. Evolution seems to have played a role.

Evolution's answer to the conflict between gender-specific reproductive strategies has been to alter reproduction such that the male of the species must exert more parental effort. The two evolutionary factors that appear to have the most impact on male reproductive strategy are uncertain paternity and hidden estrus.

While internal fertilization does create an onus of parental effort for females, it also creates the uncertainty of paternity. That is, among species with internal fertilization of the female, the male cannot simply breed, depart, and be assured of reproductive success. To ensure reproductive success, the male must remain with the female while she is fertile and prevent her from mating with other males. By doing this, the male increases the certainty of his paternity, and consequently increases his reproductive success. So, there is a trade-off: males reduce mating opportunities by staying with a specific female, yet reproductive success is increased because the male can be assured of the propagation of his offspring. This is just one manner in which evolutionary forces exert an influence on the conflicting reproductive strategies of the male and female.

While uncertain paternity exerts an influence on all species in which internal fertilization occurs, the human species is subjected to an additional evolutionary factor: hidden estrus. Estrus is the period of sexual receptivity in female mammals. In most species, the female exhibits physical signs of estrus, for example, odors, lordosis, and somatic changes. When the chimpanzee female is in estrus, her labia swells and changes colors. These visible signs of estrus serve as a signal to surrounding males of the female's sexual receptivity and the breeding begins. Among humans, visible signs of estrus have essentially disappeared. The lack of a visible sign of sexual receptivity means that the human male cannot be sure when the female is fertile and receptive. Thus the human male must maintain proximity with his mate to prevent other males from being around when she is fertile.

Concealed estrus and uncertain paternity are but two of the evolutionary forces that shape human sexual behavior. Evolution provides a prototype for a variety of other types of human sexual behavior.

Rape

Rape occurs among insects, birds, and mammals, including humans. Rape is universally perpetrated by males on females.

Thornhill (1976) described rape as it occurs in hangflies. The normal breeding ritual for this species is for the male to catch a fly and release an odor in the air. Flies are the food of the hangfly. Copulation occurs while the food is being eaten by the female. The male who is unable to procure food will sometimes try to knock a female out of the air and mate with her while she is stunned. The female typically resists, presumably in an effort to avoid accepting genes from an inadequate male.

Most birds, unlike mammals, are monogamous. Among monogamous birds living in colonies, rape is common. Studies have been conducted on ducks, swifts, herons, and gulls (Diamond 1992). It is generally recognized that among birds, males perpetrate rape on females. Rape usually occurs when the female is alone at the nest and her mate is away feeding. Females typically resist rape attempts by males. The resistance exhibited by the females appears to serve a twofold purpose: (1) to prevent mating with a male whose genes are suspect, and (2) to prevent mating that could drive away the female's current mate, thus leaving the female with all the parental responsibility.

Incest

Freud wrote about the "incest taboo," implying that it was uniquely human and that it was a sublimation of the sexual desire for blood relatives. Actually, there is little support in the field of evolution for Freud's contention that the incest taboo is a consciously derived social construct. It appears that many species naturally avoid reproduction with close blood relatives (Daly and Wilson 1983). There is good evolutionary basis to avoid inbreeding: mating among close relatives reduces fertility and reduces the survivability of offspring. Incest avoidance is evident in species as disparate as prairie dogs and rhesus monkeys (Sade 1968). Although the mechanism has not been isolated, it appears that, across many species, individuals in close proximity do not mate; those in close proximity are viewed as kin and consequently are not viewed as viable reproductive partners.

Adultery

Adultery occurs only in species that form monogamous couples. The sociobiologist views adultery as a reproductive strategy; it may be a way for an individual to increase reproductive success. The individual who has a mate yet succeeds in engendering offspring in another mate has increased his or her reproductive success. Typically, males seek adulterous sex. This makes sense, as in a monogamous species males can significantly increase reproductive success by having multiple partners, but women would not enjoy an equal increase in reproductive success. The available research does support the contention that, across human cultures, men are more interested than women in extramarital sex, men are more interested than women in having multiple sex partners, men are not selective in taking casual sex partners, and men appear to seek extramarital sex merely to obtain sexual variety (Diamond 1992).

Paraphilias

Paraphilia, or deviant sex, is culturally defined. In different cultures, different sexual acts are considered normal; a normal sexual act in one culture could be considered deviant in another. For example, Money (1988) has described the sexual practices of the Sambia people of New Guinea. In that society, prepubescent boys perform oral sex on men to obtain "men's milk." This socially mandated behavior is a cultural taboo in most other societies. Still, it is important to note that each culture may vary as to what constitutes acceptable sexual behavior. All societies have sexual prescriptions. Those who violate these standards deviate from the norm; hence, they are sexual deviants. Across species and cultures, males engage in more deviant sexual behavior than females. Unlike females, males of most species exhibit or attempt sexual behavior with members of other species, with inanimate objects, and with other unconventional mates. Although not exclusively, males are predominantly the purveyors of paraphilia.

Intercourse

Evolution has also made a tremendous impact upon the manner in which humans engage in sexual intercourse. Sexual intercourse as it has evolved does not appear to be exclusively in service of reproduction. If it were, then female fertility would not be secretive. As Diamond (1992) notes, "Whatever the main biological function of human copulation, it is not conception, which is just an occasional by-product" (p. 78). Since sexual intercourse among humans is largely unrelated to reproduction, it must serve another function. Unlike that of other animals, humans' sexual intercourse is private. The privacy of sexual intercourse and the availability for the male and female to engage in sexual intercourse even when the female is not fertile suggest that sexual intercourse among humans has evolved to serve as a means to intensify and cement monogamous relations. The pleasure derived from sexual contact in general and the orgasm in particular seems to act like classical conditioning. It builds a positive associative bond between the mates. The pleasurable aspects of sexual contact promote proximity and commitment. It would appear that among humans, sexual behavior serves as social cement.

Much information about the evolutionary influence on sexual behavior has been presented. This information can be used to understand deviant sexual behavior. Table 2–1 provides a summary of the information regarding the evolutionary influence on human sexual behavior. As can be seen, evolutionary influences appear to exert considerable influence on males to behave in a sexually deviant manner. The male reproductive strategy results in promiscuity and paraphilias. The evolutionary influences of uncertain paternity and hidden estrus have also resulted in sexual acting out by males, for example, sexual dominance. Overall, the evolutionary influences seem to promote sexual acting out by males.

Table 2–1.
Evolutionary Influence on Human Sexual Behavior

Evolutionary Factor	Human Sexual Behavior	Sexual Deviance
Male reproductive strategy	Have as many mates as possible	Promiscuity
	Select mates on superficial characteristics	Indiscriminate sex
	Sexualize unconventional sex objects	Paraphilia
Female reproductive strategy	Select mate on complex characteristics	
Uncertain paternity and hidden estrus	Males must remain with females to ensure paternity	Males try to control female and who she associates with
	Males stay with females due to uncertainty about fertility	Male tries to control female's fertility
Private sex	Intensifies sexual experience	Promotes secretiveness of sexual deviance
	Intensifies monogamous relationships	

It should be noted that just because a person's phylogenetic inheritance promotes a certain type of sexual behavior, phylogenetic inheritance cannot serve as an excuse or mitigating factor for sexual acting out. There are many behaviors that are phylogenetically influenced that are socially and legally forbidden, for example, murder. One cannot defend these other evolutionary-based behaviors and excuse them as phylogenetically determined any more than one can excuse sexual acting out as a product of evolution. People make choices and they are responsible for their choices.

Evolution is but one of the three components of the human sex drive. It does not exert influence by itself, and, like other biological components, it is modified by socialization. Evolution has caused humans to be able to innovate; perhaps this is the most uniquely human quality. Innovation is applied by humans to all aspects of evolution, for example, tool making, language, and sexual behavior. Because of innovation, knowledge about the evolutionary component of sexual behavior is important, but by itself, it contains only a fraction of what needs to be known about human sexual behavior.

Hormones

Hormones have an impact on sexual behavior in two important ways. First, hormones have an organizing influence. The hormones present during embryonic and fetal development result in permanent differentiation of sex organs. For example, the presence of testosterone during embryonic development results in male genitalia, whereas the absence of testosterone results in the development of female genitalia. Once these differences are set, they are permanent. This is how hormones exert an organizing influence. Second, hormones have an activating function. Hormones exert an influence on the mature individual, the result of which is a variety of sexual activities. Thus, hormones are said to have an activating influence; that is, hormones activate sexual behavior in the mature individual.

In humans, hormones are secreted by endocrine glands into the circulatory system. An endocrine gland is a gland that has no specialized duct for secreting its product. Instead, the gland has a rich blood supply and hormones are exported from the gland through the blood supply. Hormones are constantly being released in a small but steady stream. The flow of hormones can be influenced by such things as temperature, sunlight, stress, and diet. Hormones that do make it into the bloodstream are removed by the liver and kidneys.

Although hormones flow freely throughout the body, they do not affect all parts of the body equally. In fact, hormones really only affect target tissues, but these affected tissues may create a systemic reaction among other organs. The main function of hormones is not to create novel biological functions but to serve as catalysts and regulators of routine bodily functions.

Most of what is currently known about hormones has been discovered in the last sixty years. The first gonadal hormone was not identified until 1935. Since that time sophisticated methods have been developed to measure hormone levels. Many studies have been conducted that articulate the organizing and activating functions of hormones.

Sexual differentiation

Internal and external reproductive organs of males and females derive embryonically from the Wolffian and Müllerian ducts. Both male and female embryos have each of these ducts. In males, due to the presence of testosterone, the Wolffian duct develops into the vas deferens, seminal vesicle, testes, and prostate gland. In females, due to the lack of testosterone, the Müllerian duct develops into the ovaries, fallopian tubes, vagina, and labia. In males, since the Wolffian duct elaborates, the Müllerian duct degenerates, and the converse is true for females. All of this embryonic development occurs under the organizing influence of testosterone and other male hormones, for example, Müllerian inhibiting hormone (MIH) and dihydrotestosterone (DHT), which exert a masculinizing effect on external male genitalia.

Since sexual differentiation occurs first with internal organs and then with the external organs, variations in the hormone level can affect development. For example, if a genetic male is deprived of embryonic hormones, he will not develop male genitalia and instead appear to be female. On the other hand, if a genetic female is exposed to male hormones, she will develop external male genitalia. Thus, the presence or absence of hormones can alter the individual's genetic program.

Brain dimorphism

Males and females possess slightly different brain structures. As with internal genitalia, the male and female brain originate from a common structure, but the presence of testosterone masculinizes the male brain. It is also known that dihydrotestosterone defeminizes the male brain, further differentiating the male and female brains. The presence of masculinizing and defeminizing hormones has led researchers to believe that the converse of brain masculinization is not feminization but demasculinization and the converse of feminization is defeminization (Money 1988). Researchers speculate that because of these processes, it is possible for both masculine and feminine brain structures to coexist.

Sexual differentiation of the brain does result in some physical difference between male and female brains (Breedlove 1993). For example, it is known that the tissue that connects the two hemispheres of the brain (corpus callosum) is shaped differently in human males and females, and there is some evidence that the female's corpus callosum is proportionally larger than the male's (Utamsing and Holloway 1982). Another noteworthy difference occurs in the nucleus of the preoptic area in most mammals, which is larger in males than females (Swabb and Fliers 1985). This part of the brain is known to regulate sexual intercourse behavior in males and secretion of the luteinizing hormone in females. Differences in brain structure have also been found in the temporal lobe area with male temporal lobe asymmetry being more prominent than that found in females (Wade et al. 1985).

Brain dimorphism appears to have laid the foundation for

differences in behavior. Maccoby and Jacklin (1974) reviewed a large body of psychological studies and concluded that prominent sex differences in behavior do exist: females have better verbal ability than males; males have better visual-spatial ability than females; males have better mathematical ability than females; and in males, group dominance is more of an issue than in females.

Control of sexual behavior

The effects of hormones upon sexual behavior is partially determined by the early hormonal experience of the individual, that is, the organizing effect of embryonic and neonatal hormones. Assuming that the organizing effects of hormones have resulted in normal sexual development, then the activating effects of hormones serve to coordinate internal events, such as ovulation or sperm production, with external events, such as copulation (Carter 1993).

Sexual behaviors can be divided into three categories: motivation, courtship, and sexual intercourse. In females, hormones that cause ovulation increase sexual motivation and promote courtship behavior (Carter 1993). Estrogen appears to be the hormone that causes sexual approach behavior among female vertebrates. Estrogen also appears to increase the female's sexual attractiveness to males (Beach 1976). Copulation behavior of female mammals, or lordosis, is also influenced by the activating influence of estrogen but the organizing influence of prenatal estrogen is also critical to lordosis. Finally, it should be noted that progesterone serves to inhibit sexual motivation and it reduces courtship and copulation.

In males, testosterone appears to have its greatest impact upon sexual motivation. Low levels of testosterone, as associated with hypogonadism, appear to reduce sexual interest (Baum 1993). The impact of testosterone on copulation behavior is largely determined by embryonic and neonatal levels of testosterone experienced by the individual. With the proper exposure to testosterone early in development, it takes very little testosterone in adulthood to activate sexual behavior. Perhaps this is why castrated adult males continue to show sexual behavior for years, even decades, after castration. Sexual behavior after castration is possible because androgen production is not limited to the testes. The adrenal glands produce androgen. Furthermore, fat can act as a storehouse for hormones and, consequently, the castrated human male may have sufficient reserves for sexual behavior for many years. Testosterone appears to promote sexual interest but it is not essential to copulation behavior.

Sexual orientation

It is known that hormones can have one of four organizing effects during early development: masculinizing, demasculinizing, feminizing, and defeminizing (Money 1988). Studies with mammals reveal that exposing females to postnatal testosterone resulted in reduced sexual motivation toward males, and with prolonged exposure females showed increased sexual behavior with other females (Baum 1993). Thus, it seems possible that prenatal and postnatal exposure to varying levels of hormones may influence sexual orientation. In humans, some evidence exists to suggest that a shortage of prenatal androgens in males results only in partial brain masculinization, which is associated with homosexual orientation (Gladue et al. 1984).

Overall, it would appear that the organizing influence of hormones has a more profound effect on sexual behavior than the activating influence. Recall that the organizing influence of hormones occurs during embryonic and fetal development. The organizing influence determines the nature and quality of the development of internal and external genitalia. The organizing influence of hormones appears to play a role in sexual orientation and the selection of sexual objects. Perhaps most noteworthy is that abnormal levels of embryonic and fetal hormones can neutralize the activating influences of hormones when the individual reaches adulthood. However, the converse is not necessarily true: an individual with a normal hormonal development may be able to overcome problems in the activating influence of hormones. For example, a male castrated in adulthood is still capable of sexual behavior but a male deprived of androgen during fetal development may be incapable of normal adult sexual behavior, even if that male has normal levels of androgens as an adult. Overall, the organizing influence of hormones appears to be far more critical than the activating influence of hormones. Still the activating influence of hormones cannot be dismissed.

There is one area of sex offender treatment that does attest to the importance of activating influence of hormones. This treatment is the use of antiandrogenic agents such as medroxyprogesterone acetate. Antiandrogenic chemotherapy is used to reduce the release of androgens from the testicles. The antiandrogenic drug works by inhibiting the release of the luteinizing hormone from the pituitary gland, which in turn reduces testosterone production. The available studies indicate that use of medroxyprogesterone acetate can reduce testosterone, and consequently it can reduce frequency of sexual fantasies and arousal while increasing control over sexual urges (Berlin and Meinecke 1981, Gagne 1981). Despite the success in affecting a person's physiological and phenomenological sexual experience, antiandrogenic therapy is no panacea. Most credible antiandrogenic treatment occurs in the context of a comprehensive treatment program that includes cognitive behavioral interventions. Even in such a treatment program, use of medroxyprogesterone acetate does not necessarily assure clients of a better outcome when compared with clients who do not use such chemical agents (Meyer et al. 1992).

Hormones affect behaviors other than sexual behaviors. For example, hormones are known to play a role in parenting behavior, aggression, coping behavior, and cognitive functions (Becker et al. 1993). With regard to their influence on sexual behavior, it appears that the embryonic and neonatal influences are the most profound. It may be possible for both males and females to compensate for reduced levels of hormones in adulthood. Conversely, the absence of hormones at critical periods during early development may disrupt sexual differentiation and adulthood sexual behaviors such as sexual interest, sexual orientation, courtship, and copulation.

NEUROLOGICAL FACTORS

Paul MacLean has identified three distinct evolutionary stages in the development of the human brain (Turner 1981). As a result of this three-stage development, MacLean believes that the human brain is actually three brains in one, that is, a triunal brain. The first and the oldest of the brains is referred to as the reptilian brain. It is composed of the pons, medulla, cerebellum, and the reticular formation. This part of the brain has not been affected much by evolution, and is similar to the brain of lizards, snakes, and tortoises. Immediately above this reptilian brain is the old mammalian brain, which is largely composed of the limbic system. This part of the human brain is similar to the brain found in rats, horses, and other mammals. The third evolutionary layer of the brain is the new mammalian brain, or the neocortex. It is the part of the brain that we share with apes and monkeys, the part that is highly developed in humans and enables us to engage in uniquely human behavior, for example, abstract reasoning, creativity, and innovation.

Although the neocortex is the part of the brain that enables us to be uniquely human, it is not the part of the brain that is most associated with sexual behavior. The limbic system, part of the old mammalian brain, is the part of the brain that is most involved in sexual behavior. The word *limbic* means circular, around, or hemming in. The limbic system is a somewhat circular arrangement of certain parts of the brain. These parts of the brain are located above the hindbrain (medulla, cerebellum, and pons) and below the neocortex. Included in the limbic system are the mamillary bodies of the hypothalamus, the anterior nucleus of the thalamus, the cingulate cortex, the hippocampus, the septal nucleus, the amygdala, and some olfactory nuclei (Gazzaniga et al. 1979). The prefrontal and anterior temporal portions of the neocortex are also recognized as part of the limbic system. Equally important as the structures of the limbic system are the connections between them. It appears that connections among limbic system structures are made by the fornix, stria terminalis, and the medial forebrain bundle. These connections overlap with the Papez circuit, which has been implicated as the neurological mechanism for emotion. Overall, the limbic system is not just concerned with sexual behavior, but it has also been identified as having impact on learning, recall, emotions, and attention.

While the limbic system is clearly involved in sexual behavior, it should be recognized that other sites in the brain also play a role in determining sexual behavior. For example, McEwen (1976) discussed the fact that hormone-sensitive tissues exist throughout the brain. These tissues serve as receptor sites for gonadal hormones. Some of these receptor sites can be found in the brain stem and midbrain, which are outside the limbic system; yet they still play a role in sexual behavior.

One good method of determining the brain structures involved in sexual behavior is to study the behavior of individuals with brain pathology. Perhaps the most well-known study of sexual behavior as it relates to brain pathology was done by Klüver and Bucy (1939), who studied the behavior of monkeys with one or both of their temporal lobes ablated. Due to the contribution made by these researchers, the syndrome associated with temporal-lobe impairment is known as the Klüver-Bucy syndrome. This syndrome is characterized by damaged temporal lobes and related limbic structures, which results in hypersexuality, decreased fear and anger, increased visual stimulus–bound behavior, increased oral tendencies, and decreased ability to recognize objects.

Since Klüver and Bucy's original work, many researchers have studied the effects of temporal lobe dysfunction as it pertains to sexual behavior. Hyposexuality and hypersexuality have been noted with temporal lobe epileptics. Blumer (1970) observed that hyposexuality occurred in 59 percent of the twenty-nine temporal lobe epileptics he studied. Hyposexuality was described as limited ability to reach orgasm, infrequent sexual desire, and a low rate of sexual fantasies. Among the epileptics Blumer studied, twenty clients engaged in sexual behavior less than once a year and ten had never experienced an orgasm. Blumer suggested that the presence of chronic seizure discharges in the limbic portion of the temporal lobes resulted in decreased sexual behavior. He noted that surgical elimination of seizure focus was often associated with a dramatic increase in sexual arousal and activity. A similar phenomenon was noted after untreated clients had seizures. After a seizure, the neural activity in the limbic area decreased, and increased sexual arousal occurred.

Level of sexual arousal is but one aspect of sexual behavior affected by temporal lobe dysfunction. Ample literature exists that demonstrates that temporal lobe lesions can be associated with fetishism (Mitchell et al. 1954), transvestism (Davies and Morganstern 1960), sexual orientation (Blumer 1970), and sadism (Langevin 1990). The variety of ways in which sexual behavior is controlled by the limbic system is most evident when an individual suffers acute trauma to that area of the brain (Miller et al. 1986). Acute limbic system injury in humans has been documented to result in the following sexual behaviors: public masturbation, increased use of pornography, propositioning of male and female sexual partners, constant talk about sexual matters, pedophilia, frottage, exhibitionism, penile mutilation, and intrusive sexual fantasies.

One research team studied the effect of age of onset of temporal lobe injury (Kolarsky et al. 1967). These researchers concluded that age of onset determined the severity of the sexual problems. Specifically, they argue that temporal lobe trauma before age 3, and especially at birth, resulted in deviant sexual behavior such as voyeurism, exhibitionism, leg fetishism, sadism, frotteurism, masochism, and pedophilia. On the other hand, temporal lobe trauma after age 3 resulted in a lower incidence of sexual deviation. The researchers speculated that an early brain lesion destroys primordial programs controlling the selection of viable sexual objects and activities.

The foregoing literature is based upon case studies of clinical populations. The subjects in these studies presented with neurological problems and it was discovered that they also engaged in deviant sexual behavior. But what about those studies that select subjects because they have been arrested for a sexual offense? In these studies subjects are identified first for their deviant sexual behavior, and then neurological examinations are conducted.

Neurological and neuropsychological examination of adult sex offenders has been discussed in the literature for many years. Yet there is little definitive information and a consensus seems to be far away. Two problems plague this research. First, there is the problem of classifying sex offenders. As a group, sex offenders are heterogeneous. It is known that one sex offender may engage in a variety of paraphilias (Abel et al. 1988). This makes classification of sex offenders based upon type of behavior unreliable. It is also known that one sex offender can attack both children and adults, males and females (Abel et al. 1987). So classification of sex offenders based upon victim characteristics is unreliable.

Even classification of offenders using the plethysmograph is unreliable (Adams et al. 1992). The second problem plaguing the neurological study of sex offenders is the problem of measurement. Presently, there are no agreed-upon standard neurological measures for sexual behavior. In fact, there are those who argue that at this time we do not even know which techniques are best suited to identify the brain structures and functions associated with sexual deviance (Langevin et al. 1989). Attempts have been made to use simultaneous, multiple neurological and neuropsychological measures in an attempt to fully articulate brain structure and function. Still, problems emerge because of the lack of agreement among multiple measures. Contradictory and inconsistent results from different measures are difficult to interpret, but they do not come as a complete surprise. Tsushima and Wedding (1979) compared diagnostic conclusions of the Halstead-Reitan test with CT scans and found agreement in only 56 percent of the cases. Some researchers rather optimistically contend that the varying results of assessment techniques does not mean that the results are contradictory, but rather that the results are complementary and reflect differing specificity of the measurements (Hucker et al. 1988). While this contention may be true, the problem of reconciling inconsistent results of multiple measures still remains unresolved.

It is important to recognize the aforementioned limitations regarding neurological research with sex offenders, but that is not to imply that no useful research exists on the topic. Good empirical neurological and neuropsychological research regarding sex offenders has been ongoing for at least four decades. Some of the more noteworthy studies published in the last ten years are presented in Table 2–2.

Even though Table 2–2 presents test results for subtypes of sex offenders, it may be prudent to combine the results of these subtypes of sex offenders and look at differences between sex offenders and controls. Recall that it is difficult to classify sex offenders with a great deal of reliability. In taking this approach, a consistent finding seems to emerge: sex offenders perform more poorly on neuropsychological tests and exhibit more abnormalities on neurological examinations as compared with controls. The reason for this finding is not immediately evident. The neurological impairment and abnormality observed among sex offenders could have occurred for a variety of reasons. While the etiology of these problems remains unknown, one evident finding emerges: a subset of sex offenders has identifiable neurological impairment.

As mentioned above, it may not be prudent to look at the subtypes of sex offenders as listed in Table 2–2. For example, some authors identified violent and nonviolent sex offenders for the purposes of comparison (Galski et al. 1990, Hucker et al. 1988). Such classifications may be inaccurate because sex offenders typically engage in more than one type of paraphilia, and a sex offender who appears violent during one act may be nonviolent when engaging in a different paraphilia act. Furthermore, sex offenders who select a child as a victim are also known to sexually victimize adults as well (Abel et al. 1987).

Given that it may be premature to begin teasing apart various neurological impairments as associated with specific paraphilias, the information in Table 2–2 can still be used to detect general trends in the research findings. Consider the following:

- Sex offenders exhibit low-average intelligence.
- Sex offenders exhibit abnormality in the left temporal lobe, which may account for the finding of weak verbal skills.
- Sex offenders exhibit right hemisphere abnormalities, which may be related to the finding that sex offenders are below average in social perception, social problem solving, and synthetic reasoning skills.

Table 2-2.
Summary of Findings of Physiological and Neuropsychological Assessment of Sex Offenders

Type of Offender	WAIS-R	Halstead-Reitan or Lauria-Nebraska	CT Scan	Findings
Langevin et al. 1989				
Pedophile, same sex victims (PS), (n=50)	PS/FSIQ=90 PO/FSIQ=93 PE/FSIQ=105 Control=104	PS Impair Index = .35 PO Impair Index = .26 PE Impair Index = .34 Control Impair Index = .17 (Halstead-Reitan)	44% PS Abnormal 33% PO Abnormal 22% PE Abnormal 34 Control Abnormal	• PS & PO have lower IQ scores than Controls • PO & PE have more impairment than PS or Controls • PO may have left hemisphere impairment • Verbal skills low for PS and PO
Pedophile, opposite sex victim (PO), (n=50)				
Pedophile, either sex victim (PE), (n=50)				
Control (n=36)				
Langevin et al. 1988				
Incest Offender (n=91) Control (n=36) (Non-violent, non-sex offending criminals)	Incest/FSIQ=95 Control/FSIQ=107	13% Incest Impairment No Control Impairment (Halstead-Reitan)	24% Incest Impaired 30% Control Impaired	• Intelligence average for incest group • Incest has less social awareness and attention to detail as compared to Control (Picture Arrg. & Compl)

| Hucker et al. 1988 | Sadists (SAD), (n = 22) Non-Sadist Sex Offender (NONSAD), (n = 21) Control (n = 36) (Non-violent, non-sex offender criminal) | .54% Impaired SAD and NONSAD combined 16% Controls Impaired (Lauria-Nebraska) | 50% SAD Abnormal 39% NONSAD Abnormal 36% Control Abnormal | •Incest has lower abstract reasoning ability (Category Test) •Violent incest offenders show temporal lobe abnormality •Victim-offender not biologically related correlated with more CT abnormalities •Sadists show more abnormalities than other two groups (CT Scan) •Right temporal horn frequently dilated in sadist (CT Scan) •Non-sadistic offenders show global, nonlateralized impairment |

(continued)

Table 2-2.
(Continued)

	Type of Offender	WAIS-R	Halstead-Reitan or Lauria-Nebraska	CT Scan	Findings
Scott et al. 1985	Adult Rapist (AR), (n=21) Pedophile (Ped), (n=18) Control (n=38) (Hospitalized and non-hospitalized volunteers)		AR Pathognomic Score = 42 Ped Pathognomic Score = 57 (Lauria-Nebraska)		• Pedophiles show more impairments than rapists or controls
Hucker et al. 1986	Pedophiles (n=39) Controls (n=14) (Non-sex, non-violent offenders)	PED/FSIQ=97 Control/FSIQ=107	37% Pedophiles Impaired 17% Controls Impaired	52% Pedophiles Abnormal 17% Controls Abnormal	• Although pedophile average FSIQ is normal, there are many in lower range • Pedophiles show more impairment than Controls on neurological test • Pedophiles show dilation of temporal and anterior horns

Study	Subjects	Results	Conclusions
Hendricks et al. 1988	Child Molester (n=16) Control (n=16) (University staff, all control were female)	• Child molesters lower blood flow compared to Controls • Child molesters have thinner and less dense skulls than Controls	• All results suggest pedophiles have more temporal-parietal abnormalities • Blood flow of child molesters is indicative of pathological status
Galski et al. 1990	Violent Sex Offender (V), (n=21) Non-violent Sex Offender (NV), (n=14) Control	49% of all sex offenders show impairment 65% of violent sex offenders show impairment 35% of NV sex offenders show impairment (Lauria-Nebraska)	• Violent sex offenders were predicted by left hemisphere and left sensory-motor impairments • Violent offenders show impairment in expressive speech • Non-violent offenders show impairment in the right parietal-occipital and left frontal regions

While these trends in the data amount to a modest beginning in the effort to understand the neurological basis of deviant sexual behavior, it is a beginning nonetheless. It is a foundation upon which future research can build. Hopefully, research in other areas will be used to corroborate efforts to uncover the neurological foundation of sexual deviance. For example, much research has been done that identifies two types of aggression—reactive and predatory. Also, a considerable body of literature exists regarding endocrine, neurotransmitters, brain wave, and neuroanatomical factors associated with aggression (Meloy 1988). Another area of research that might contribute to our understanding of the neurological basis of sexual deviance is the research pertaining to psychopaths. Once again, a considerable body of literature exists regarding the biological and neurological factors associated with psychopathy (Hart et al. 1990). This literature may also prove useful in furthering our quest to uncover the neurological basis of deviant sexual behavior.

The three biological factors that constitute the human sex drive are evolutionary, hormonal, and neurological. The literature reviewed in this section shows how disruption in one of these areas can result in abnormal sexual behavior. Based upon this finding, it can be argued that deviation in the human sex drive can result in deviations in sexual behavior. However, this is not the full picture. Socialization and disinhibition also play determining roles in deviant sexual behavior.

SOCIALIZATION

In the context of the proposed etiological theory, socialization refers to learning sexual behavior. The primary effect of socialization is to enable the individual to acquire an internalized plan of socially acceptable sexual behavior. Freud's notion of id, ego, and superego provides a handy metaphor for the socialization process: the human sex drive (id) must be shaped so that it enables the person to engage in appropriate sexual behavior (ego) in a responsible manner (superego).

Biological factors play a tremendous role in determining socialization. Evolutionary factors influence sex roles. Hormonal factors influence sexual interest and motivation, which in turn affect the types of behaviors an individual learns. Neurological factors affect attention, memory, concentration, comprehension, and probably the selection of sexual objects. Overall, it must be recognized that the sex drive exerts influence on socialization. If the sex drive is normal, then the individual has a good chance of learning normal sexual behaviors. Abnormalities in the sex drive can exert an influence that results in the individual learning abnormal or deviant sexual behavior.

Socialization by itself can play a determining role in sexual behavior. While the research has found neurological abnormalities among sex offenders (Table 2–2), not all sex offenders were identified as neurologically impaired. This suggests that less than 100 percent of all sex offenders are neurologically impaired. Actually, it is likely that 30 to 60 percent of sex offenders have some neurological impairment. So what of the sex offenders who do not have neurological impairment? Why do they exhibit deviant behavior? The answer is, socialization. These individuals are socialized in such a manner that they learn deviant sexual behavior. Thus, socialization appears to be the pathway through which biologically normal individuals come to exhibit deviant sexual behavior.

Socialization of the sex drive occurs at two levels. First, the individual must be socialized with respect to cognitive factors that control and shape expression of the sexual drive. The cognitive factors that play such a role include beliefs, values, and expectations regarding sexual behavior. Second, socialization results in the individual acquiring a set of behaviors that makes sexual behavior viable in a particular social context. That is, a person learns courtship and mating behavior as a result of socialization. This section discusses the socialization factors of cognitive controls and behavior patterns.

Cognitive Factors

Bem (1970) defines a belief as the perceived relationship between two things. He notes that a belief system has a hierarchical structure: basic beliefs, called zero-order beliefs, are combined to create more complex beliefs, for example, first-order beliefs. Bem defines attitudes as likes and dislikes, an affinity for or an aversion to specific situations, objects, persons, groups, ideas, or philosophies. Attitudes, like beliefs, can be arranged hierarchically. Attitudes are different from beliefs in that attitudes carry a significant emotional component, whereas beliefs are largely intellectual. Values are thought to be a subset, or certain type, of attitude. Bem contends that beliefs and attitudes have a reciprocal relationship with behavior: beliefs and attitudes influence our behavior and our behavior can cause us to modify and alter our beliefs and attitudes.

Beliefs and attitudes are important to our understanding of behavior, and sexual behavior in particular, because people strive to maintain consistency among beliefs, attitudes, and behaviors. When behavior is inconsistent with beliefs and attitudes, the individual experiences dissonance (Festinger 1957). Dissonance is uncomfortable and creates anxiety, which in turn creates motivation for individuals to either change their behavior or modify their attitudes and beliefs. Thus, it is apparent that there is a reciprocal interaction between attitudes and beliefs, and behavior. Furthermore, it can be argued that if one knows an individual's beliefs and attitudes, to some extent one can anticipate the range of behavior exhibited by that individual.

The relationship of cognitive factors and sexually deviant behavior has been explored. In particular, a wealth of research regarding the beliefs and expectations of sex offenders exists. This literature spans almost forty years. A summary of four decades of research pertaining to the cognitions of sex offenders is provided in Table 2-3. Most of the research differentiates between child molesters and rapists. Some noteworthy trends in the data regarding these two types of offenders appear to emerge.

The research summarized in Table 2-3 reveals that child molesters and rapists differ in terms of their cognitions. Rapists appear similar to males in the general population with regard to attitudes, but rapists tend to be hyposensitive to cues that indicate a person may be experiencing discomfort or anxiety. On the other hand, the research suggests that child molesters are hypersensitive to social cues, but they interpret these cues so that they expect rejection and hostility. In general, child molesters have low self-confidence, rigid values, expectations that interactions with adults will be unrewarding, and expectations that interactions with children will be rewarding. Overall, it would appear that child molesters hold beliefs that promote sexual contact with children, whereas rapists tend to be aware of socially acceptable beliefs but they may be unaware of when these beliefs are in conflict with their behavior.

The issue of sex offenders incorrectly perceiving others has long been discussed by treatment providers. Most recently, Yochelson and Samenow (1976) identified specific ways in which criminals perceive the world differently than noncriminals. Since the criminal perceptions were deemed to be a distorted view of reality, the criminal perceptual and thinking patterns have become known as thinking errors. Today, it is rare when a sex offender treatment provider does not use the concept of thinking errors in planning and executing treatment. In fact, the elimination of thinking errors is viewed as a primary goal in most sex offender

Table 2-3.
Cognitive Factors Characteristic of Child Molesters and Rapists

Researcher(s)	Findings
Hammer and Glueck 1957	Based upon Thematic Apperception Test (TAT) results, they conclude child molesters fear heterosexual contact.
Frisbie et al. 1967	Based upon semantics differential, child molesters do not believe they fulfill role expectations in social interactions.
Gebhart et al. 1965	Child molesters advocate strong moral values against premarital sex. Child molesters are described as being rigid moralists.
Goldstein et al. 1973	Child molesters report more guilt and shame from looking at pornography than do rapists or controls.
Howells 1978	Child molesters view children as nonthreatening and positive, whereas adults are viewed as domineering.
Fields 1978	Persons who maintain traditional sex role expectations tend to blame women for rape.
Segal and Stermac 1984	Rapists do not necessarily endorse traditional sex roles for women. Lower socioeconomic males tend to have sex role expectations similar to rapists.
Segal and Marshall 1985	In videotaped interactions with females, higher socioeconomic males are more assertive than other males. Analysis of role play scenarios does not uncover social deficits in rapists, but child molesters are identified as less assertive.
Overholser and Beck 1986	Administered questionnaires regard sexual attitudes, social distress, social rejection, and rape myths; discovered no difference among rapists, non-sex offender criminals, low-socioeconomic subjects, and persons with limited dating experience. Comparisons of child molesters to other subjects revealed child molesters expect social rejection.
Lipton et al. 1987	Using videotape recordings of social interactions, rapists are discovered to be deficient in correctly interpreting social cues; for example, rapists have difficulty recognizing a female's nonverbal cues of distress and discomfort.
Segal and Stermac 1990	Child molesters differ from other groups regarding interpretation of stories of sexual contact between adults and children. Child molesters tend to perceive such sexual contact as less harmful, more beneficial, and less in need of sanctions than controls.

treatment programs. Although practitioners regularly use the concept of thinking errors, it has not often been the subject of empirical study (Lanyon 1986). Still, the research that has focused on this issue has had no difficulty in discovering and identifying thinking errors (Neidigh and Krop 1992). Ultimately, the real issue may be not identifying thinking errors, but organizing thinking errors into a coherent system or nomenclature.

For the most part, the available evidence suggests that sex offenders display cognitions that promote sexual deviance. These cognitions may come in the form of expectations that deviant sexual contact is preferable; for example, the child molester's view of adults as domineering and children as positive. Or the cognitions may be distorted, and action based upon the distorted beliefs will result in unacceptable sexual behavior. In general, the role of cognitions in determining sexual behavior is clear: thought precedes action, and deviant thoughts precede deviant sexual behavior.

Behavior Patterns

In most species, each individual conforms to a uniform courtship and mating pattern that is phylogenetically determined (Money 1988). In humans, mating and courtship is influenced by one's culture, community, and family. As a result, human courtship and mating behavior is only partially determined by phylogenetic influences. Humans show a great deal of individual variation in sexual behavior. Still, humans have not become entirely liberated from evolutionary influences. Vestiges of phylogenetic sexual behavior is still evident among humans.

Daly and Wilson (1983) discuss the phylogenetic influence on courtship behaviors of humans in a variety of cultures. They begin with the observation, that across cultures, husbands are older than their wives. They argue that this is quite understandable when reproductive success is considered as a determining factor. They state that if it is important to maximize reproductive potential, then a man could hardly do better than to seek a healthy young female. Conversely, the female should not select a male for his youth or appearance, but for the resources he commands. Wealth, belongings, and success identify the man with the most resources to devote to parenting. Such resources take time to acquire, and consequently females would do well to select older males.

Other authors tend to support this notion that evolutionary forces do influence sexual behavior patterns among humans. For example, Coombs and Kenkel (1966) surveyed men and women participating in a computer dating service. They discovered that women sought mates who were intelligent, high status, stable, and of similar religious beliefs. Men sought mates who had good qualities, but whereas women were not insistent that their mates be attractive, men rated physical attractiveness as an important quality. Furthermore, women were choosier after dates, and they rated their dates as "marriage material" far less often than males.

So, if humans do follow phylogenetic blueprints for courtship and mating behavior, what is the evolutionary mechanism that serves as the blueprint? Diamond (1992) argues that we have search images, mental images against which we compare objects and people around us in order to be able to recognize something quickly. Diamond states that we have search images for mates, and that is why married couples are very similar with regard to religion, race, socioeconomic status, personality, and intelligence. As might be expected, spouses are least similar on physical characteristics, but the research does suggest that we select mates with whom we share some physical characteristics—all the way to the length of one's earlobe.

Money (1988) has taken the concept of search image and amplified it. In his schema, search image is referred to as a lovemap—a personalized, developmental representation that depicts an idealized lover and an idealized program of sexual behavior. Money states that everyone has a lovemap and each person's lovemap is as unique as one's fingerprints. It appears that a person's lovemap is particularly useful in the courtship phase. Courtship is viewed as a sequence of behaviors that follows a specific order: establishing contact, verbal interaction, closer proximity, body to body contact, orifice contact, and intromitting. While each individual is free to innovate and maintain his/her own unique lovemap, all lovemaps contain the aforementioned components. In addressing the issue of paraphilia, Money explains that for one to engage in a paraphilic act, he/she must first have a paraphilic lovemap. Money identifies forty paraphilias and states that there is a lovemap for each.

There is research that supports the contention that sex offenders have a personalized pattern of sexual behavior unique to themselves. For years, law enforcement personnel have identified the work of serial rapists by their modus operandi. The concept of modus operandi has a counterpart in the clinical literature. Those professionals conducting treatment with sex offenders have used the concept of the offense cycle, a characteristic pattern of behavior that includes antecedent and consequential behaviors engaged in by the offender (Ferrara 1992). It has been widely recognized that sex offenders do exhibit idiosyncratic patterns of sexual behavior. The concepts of lovemaps and search images help explain why the sex offender's behavior is so consistent across time and in different situations: the offender follows his lovemap and consequently tends to repeat the same type of acts over and over.

Applying the notion that sex offenders use an unacceptable lovemap to determine courtship behaviors, the two most frequently discussed paraphilias — rape and child molesting — can be reexamined. In the context of the lovemap, rape can be defined as an offender omitting initial courtship behaviors (e.g., verbal interaction, proximity, body to body contact) and moving straight to intromitting, against the victim's explicit feedback that such contact is undesired. Child molesting can be construed as use of all the appropriate steps of courtship, but selecting a mate that is inappropriate due to age. The behaviors that professionals view as "grooming" have their context in a lovemap, and these behaviors fall under the activities of establishing contact, verbal interaction, and closer proximity. In general, using the concept of lovemaps or search images tends to make deviant sexual behavior more comprehensible; sexual deviance is an unacceptable variation on a socially acceptable pattern of sexual behavior.

Finally, if paraphiliacs have paraphilic lovemaps, it would be reasonable to expect that the paraphiliac would not possess a normal lovemap. Consequently, the paraphiliac would not be expected to be particularly good at engaging in normative sexual behavior. This is consistent with the current literature that identifies child molesters as lacking in heterosocial skills (Segal and Marshall 1985) and rapists as lacking in recognition of social cues exhibited by females (Lipton et al. 1987).

Socialization is a key factor in the explanation of deviant sexual behavior. Since socialization affects both the cognitive and behavioral repertoire of the individual, clues to understanding deviant sexual behavior need to be sought in each of these domains. The existing literature offers some insights regarding how sex offenders think and behave. In general, it would appear that the literature indicates that sexual deviants behave as they do because their beliefs, expectations, and cognitions support this type of behavior.

DISINHIBITION

The concept of disinhibition is useful in developing an understanding of temporal and situational factors associated with acting out by paraphiliacs. Disinhibition is the process of unleashing or liberating thoughts, desires, or behaviors that an individual had consciously tried to control or eliminate. The process of trying to control or eliminate a behavior is inhibition. The process of relinquishing control is disinhibition.

Some work has been done to identify the process of disinhibition as it relates to sexual acting out. In fact, specific disinhibitors that act as precursors to sexually deviant behavior have been identified (Pithers et al. 1988). This research suggests that the disinhibitors for rapists and child molesters differ. Consider the rank ordered list of disinhibitors for rapists and pedophiles in Table 2-4.

Inspection of Table 2-4 reveals that rapists and child molesters have only one disinhibitor in common: low self-esteem. This suggests that for both rapists and child molesters, the deviant sexual act may be a means of managing and bolstering self-esteem. The bulk of the disinhibitors for rapists look vaguely familiar as the prominent emotional features of an antisocial personality, that is, anger and thrill seeking. The disinhibitors for the child molester are consistent with previously discussed research that describes these offenders as timid, undersocialized, and fearful.

It is interesting to note that alcohol and drug abuse are not listed as disinhibitors. That does not mean that substance abuse cannot be a disinhibitor. Alcohol or drug abuse does occur in a minority of cases of sexual offenses. According to Pithers and colleagues (1988), many offenders engage in careful planning to make it appear as if their acts were

Table 2-4.
Rank Order of Disinhibitors for Rapists and Child Molesters

Rapists	Child Molesters
Generalized anger	Deviant sexual plans
Anger toward women	Low self-esteem
Opportunity	Deviant sexual fantasies
Low self-esteem	Generalized anxiety
Boredom	Social anxiety

unplanned. To the extent that chemical abuse can serve as subterfuge, the sex offender will use it.

Finkelhor and colleagues (1986) have examined the disinhibition literature as it relates to child molesting. Like Pithers and colleagues (1988), they believe that alcohol may be used by an offender to enable him to do what he wants to do, that is, commit a sex offense. They suggest that the role of disinhibition in the commission of child molestation has some empirical support. Specifically, the research indicates that pedophiles are individuals with poor impulse control: they fail to inhibit impulses that another person may readily eliminate or rechannel. Thus, disinhibition appears to play a role in some sexual acting out by child molesters.

In general, it would appear that disinhibition does play a role in the manifestation of deviant sexual behavior. Among fully socialized individuals, a disinhibitor may prompt sexual acting out. Among paraphiliacs, a disinhibitor may be the trigger for their offense cycle.

CONCLUSIONS

The proposed etiological model of sexual deviance is quite comprehensive. To the extent that it accounts for and integrates much of the existing knowledge abut sex offenders, it is a good model. Like any other model, the proposed model should be able to make predictions about the behavior of sex offenders, and these predictions should be consistent with the existing research. Consider the following list of predictions derived from each of the components of the model theory:

Evolution

- Males will engage in deviant sex more often than females.

- Females will be victims of deviant sex more often than males.
- Given the male's propensity to be less selective about mating behavior, more males than females will engage in adultery, multiple partners, fetishism, and transvestism.

Hormones

- Maternal health can affect fetal hormonal levels, and as a result, sexual orientation, sexual interest, and sexual motivation can be affected.
- Castration will not prevent an individual from engaging in deviant or appropriate sexual behavior.

Neurological Factors

- Abnormalities in the limbic system, temporal lobes, or prefrontal areas may result in deviant sexual behavior.
- The earlier in the individual's life that a neurological abnormality occurs, the more disrupted and deviant the sexual behavior will be.
- Since the neural structures involved in emotion and sexual behavior overlap, it is possible that strong emotions (e.g., anger) can activate deviant sexual behavior.

Socialization

- Sex offenders display cognitions that support their deviant sexual desires. These cognitions are at such a variance with normal social perceptions that they can be referred to as cognitive distortions.
- Child molesters tend to view interactions with children as more positive than interactions with adults. Sexual

contact with children is but one aspect of the child molester's preference for children as opposed to adults.

- Rapists can be identified by a perceptual insensitivity or a cognitive ignorance of social cues.
- Everyone develops a schema to guide his/her sexual behavior, and paraphilic behavior is guided by a paraphilic schema.
- Each individual has a characteristic pattern of sexual behavior, and among sex offenders this pattern is known as the offense cycle.

Disinhibition

- Normal individuals may engage in paraphilic behavior in the presence of disinhibitors.
- Sex offenders are more likely to engage in deviant sexual behavior when they are disinhibited.
- Different disinhibitors exist for different types of sex offenders.

To a large extent the predictions based upon the proposed model are consistent with existing research. It is important to note that although this model of the etiology of sexual deviance began in an attempt to understand the neurologically impaired sex offender, the proposed model actually pertains to all sex offenders. This model can be used to explain the deviant sexual behavior of persons with and without neurological impairment. The model applies to low IQ and high IQ offenders, offenders from different cultures, female offenders, and persons with a wide variety of paraphilias, for example, fetishism or transvestism.

Perhaps the most important feature of this proposed model is that it provides a context for understanding a great deal of our existing knowledge about sexual behavior. This is a book about treating the neurologically and psychiatrically impaired sex offender. As often happens in a book about a specialty topic, the issue of neuropathy or psychopathology could be elevated to a monolithic explanatory factor. That error will not be made in this book. The issues of neuropathy and psychopathology are important but these factors have a context. The context for these factors is the biological sex drive and the socialization process. The proposed model affords the opportunity to integrate these issues into the existing knowledge about normal and deviant sexual behavior. The result will be, it is hoped, a deeper understanding of the issues and more effective treatment.

3

Neuropsychological Essentials: Modification to Traditional Treatment

Persons with neurological impairment are different. They are different from how they were prior to their brains being compromised. They are different from people without such impairments in many respects, including memory, concentration, attention, and higher-order cognitive functions. Because persons with neurological impairments are different, the approach that one takes in treating them should also be different. The focus of this chapter is to discuss the ways in which treatment of juvenile sex offenders with neurological problems differs from treatment of nonimpaired sex offenders. This chapter is divided into two sections. In the first section a general strategy for treating the neurologically impaired client will be discussed. In the second section specific guidelines for intervention with the neurologically impaired juvenile sex offender are provided. Taken together the general strategy and the specific guidelines are intended to help clinicians conduct treatment with the neurologically impaired juvenile sex offender.

GENERAL STRATEGY

The mere thought of doing therapy with the neurologically impaired juvenile sex offender may be daunting. It is likely

that many clinicians who face this challenge will feel per-
plexed. While it is prudent to know one's limitations, it is
useful to realize that some of the standard training that most
clinicians receive does in fact prepare them to begin work with
the neurologically impaired juvenile sex offender. In this section, two issues pertaining to the treatment of neurologically
impaired juvenile sex offenders are discussed: first, the personality of the neurologically impaired client will be compared
to the primitive personality. Second, a method for structuring
treatment of neurologically impaired clients is presented. This
treatment approach is based upon the recognition that the
neurologically impaired client has difficulty acquiring and
generalizing new skills. Overall, this discussion is intended to
provide a framework for understanding and working with the
neurologically impaired juvenile sex offender.

Organic Personality

One of the most fundamental divisions in our current
diagnostic system is the division between organic and functional diagnoses. Miller (1992) argues that this division may
not be as inviolate as it might appear in textbooks. Specifically, Miller suggests that the cognitive style of primitive
personalities has a basis in the way that their brains are
organized, and this brain organization is similar to that of
persons with organic personalities. Consequently, it is suggested that persons with primitive personalities are similar
neurologically and psychologically to persons with neurological impairments.

It is difficult to distinguish the primitive personality from
the neurologically impaired person based on the listing of
personality descriptors. Consider the following list of shared
features of primitive and organic personalities:

- Lack of personality integration.
- Limited ability to modulate and control emotions.

- Tendency to become bound to the immediate situation.
- Limited ability to sustain stable attachments.
- Behavior tends to be impulsive.
- Relationships tend to be destructive.
- The person may feel unreal and detached from surrounding events.
- Interpersonal boundaries are not respected.
- Lack of integration of emotions and cognitions.

Is this a list of attributes of the primitive personality, the neurologically impaired person, or both? It actually describes both the primitive and the organic personalities. As Miller (1992) suggests, there may be more than mere surface similarities between these two diagnostic categories. There may also be underlying etiological commonalities, for example, brain injury or brain organization.

The issue of shared etiological commonalities may warrant some amplification as it is unorthodox to suggest etiological similarities between functional and organic diagnostic categories. In the preceding chapter the neuropsychological research regarding sex offenders was discussed. It was noted that there is little agreement between neuropsychological tests and physiological measures of functioning. It may be possible that some sex offenders do poorly on neuropsychological tests because of the way that their brains are organized, not because they have suffered a brain injury. It is known that many sex offenders who may be classified as neurologically impaired on neuropsychological tests have never suffered a brain injury. Thus, one can function in a manner similar to a brain-injured person even without suffering a brain injury. This is precisely Miller's contention regarding the common etiological basis of the primitive and organic personalities: the organization of the brain of the primitive personality is similar to the injured brain in the organic personality disorder.

Based upon the shared behavioral characteristics of the

organic and primitive personalities, and the possibility of shared etiological factors, it seems appropriate to consider using similar therapeutic techniques for these problems. It may be that interventions and strategies that are effective with primitive personalities may also be effective with the neurologically impaired client (Robbins 1989). Consider the following general guidelines for intervention with the primitive personality that may also apply to the neurologically impaired client:

1. The goal of treatment should be to increase self-control. Treatment should not focus on delving into the past. Examination of past trauma may elicit strong emotions that could disorganize the individual.
2. The focus of treatment should be upon behavior that occurs in the here and now. The client should strive to increase self-awareness about current behaviors that may be problematic. Increased awareness of problem behaviors should result in plans and efforts for increased control.
3. It is important to discuss the client's disability and resulting impairments in functioning. The client needs to have a realistic assessment of his/her capabilities. Clients may find it easy to admit to simple or concrete impairments, for example, neglect of a body part. Clients may find it more difficult to be aware of higher-order cognitive impairments; the skill that is necessary for self-awareness may be one of the skills that are diminished by the impairments.
4. Provide an explanatory model for treatment. Included in this explanatory model must be an explanation of how the client's disability affects treatment. Clients will need to understand treatment if they are to become active participants in the treatment process.

A general theme permeates these recommendations: the clinician should prepare the client and limit the scope of treatment. The clinician should support the client's sense of self before embarking upon the change process. The change process should be limited and focus largely upon the client's present behavior; that is, the goal of treatment is to alter the client's current pattern of behavior.

Learning

Neurologically impaired persons learn more slowly than persons without such impairments. The learning that does occur seems to disintegrate more quickly. There tends to be limited ability to generalize learning or transfer skills beyond the setting in which the learning occurred. Given such difficulties it comes as no surprise that few clinicians choose to work with neurologically impaired clients, especially neurologically impaired juvenile sex offenders.

The problems associated with memory and learning impairments are real but they are not insurmountable. Toglia (1991) has proposed a multicontext approach for treating persons with brain injuries. In this approach, it is assumed that clients will have difficulty acquiring and generalizing new skills and information. To remedy this problem, Toglia recommends an approach based upon four components: use of multiple environments, metacognitive training, combining new and existing knowledge, and processing strategies. Each component of Toglia's approach is defined and discussed below.

Use of multiple environments. Transfer entails differentiating a skill or strategy from the environment in which it was learned and applying it in a new situation. If a skill or strategy becomes overidentified to a specific environment, that skill or strategy will never be used in other environments. Conversely, if a person learns to use skills in a variety of situations, the person is less bound by environment.

Transfer is not an all-or-nothing phenomenon. Transfer occurs along a continuum:

Near transfer—The learning environment and the new situation share all but one or two characteristics.

Intermediate transfer—The learning environment and the new environment share only a few common characteristics.

Far transfer—The new environment shares no surface characteristic with the learning environment, that is, the two environments are conceptually similar but not physically similar.

An appropriate goal for transfer training with head-injured persons is intermediate transfer. Far transfer is clearly the most desirable goal but it may not always occur with neurologically impaired clients.

Metacognitive training.   This therapeutic component refers to training designed to increase self-awareness and self-critical evaluation. There are those who contend that meaningful transfer can only occur if metacognitive skills exist (Belmont et al. 1982). The problem frequently encountered with persons who suffer brain injuries is that self-awareness is often impaired. In fact, persons with brain injuries frequently underestimate the severity of their disability and the impact that it has on their functioning.

Decreased self-awareness is problematic in two ways. First, the lack of self-awareness reduces corrective feedback, that is, the person is unaware that he or she is making mistakes. Second, the lack of awareness of impaired functioning decreases the likelihood that a person will use compensatory skills or strategies. After all, there is no need to compensate if a deficit does not exist. Both of these obstacles prevent the brain-injured person from correcting mistakes and learning from experience.

There are specific techniques that can enhance metacognitive skills. Consider the following methods of metacognitive training:

Feedback — A therapist provides feedback to the person regarding performance. For feedback to be instructive, the therapist should identify the specific mistakes the person made that resulted in poor performance.

Self-estimation — The person predicts success or accuracy in completing a task before the task is undertaken. Afterward, the person compares performance with prediction. The objective is to increase the accuracy of predictions.

Role reversal — The therapist adopts the role of the person. The therapist performs a task, making errors that the person must identify. The goal is to increase error detection.

Self-question — At specific times during a task, the person is asked to stop and answer two or three standard questions, such as, "How am I doing?" "Am I doing what I should?" and "Am I following directions?"

Self-evaluation — After performing an activity, the person fills out a questionnaire designed to accurately assess outcome.

The metacognitive training techniques assume that the person does have difficulty with self-awareness. These techniques are designed to enhance self-awareness. If these techniques are used repetitively, then the techniques may help compensate for memory impairments.

Combining new and existing information. Information is learned more rapidly and is more easily retained when it is associated with existing information. If new information is perceived as abstract or irrelevant, the person has difficulty learning. Conversely, if the information is related to previous experiences, learning occurs more rapidly.

There are two techniques that can be used to facilitate associations between new and existing information:

Similarity training — The counselor provides instruction to the person regarding the various environments in which a skill or strategy would be useful. The counselor emphasizes that the skill or strategy can be used in similar situations.

Cue identification — The counselor helps the person to develop a list of cues that signal the appropriateness of a skill or strategy. In essence, the person is taught to use the skill or strategy when specific cues are recognized.

These techniques are particularly powerful in facilitating transfer of training. They are useful with persons who have cognitive impairments.

Processing strategies. Information processing refers to the manner in which a person collects, analyzes, and responds to information. The person with a brain injury has difficulty processing information. The basis of this difficulty is often the result of weak or nonexistent strategies for processing information. Thus, one point of intervention for the neurologically impaired client is to teach new processing strategies.

There are two types of processing strategies that appear to have some utility with brain-injured clients (Toglia 1991):

Situational strategies — Strategies designed to be effective in a particular environment or situation, for example, rehearsal and practice of a desired behavior.

Nonsituational strategies — Information-processing strategies that apply to multiple situations or environments, for example, planning ahead or self-monitoring.

Each strategy has its utility. Situational strategies are effective when the behavior being taught is appropriate for situations that occur on a routine basis, such as meals, grooming, greetings, or travel. On the other hand, it is not possible to prepare for every situation, especially situations that occur rarely. In these instances, the nonsituational strategies will be most effective.

Overall, learning and transfer of learning can be enhanced by Toglia's multicontext approach. Each component of this approach is designed to address learning deficits that are frequently encountered when working with neurologically impaired clients. By themselves, each of the four components of this approach provides the basis for creating powerful interventions with neurologically impaired clients. When all four components are used in combination throughout treatment, learning and generalization can occur.

Taken in tandem, the guidelines generated based upon the primitive personality and the structure inherent in the multicontext approach provide a good framework for developing an organized treatment strategy for the neurologically impaired juvenile sex offender. The confluence of these two treatment domains indicates that an effective strategy for the neurologically impaired juvenile sex offender is one that focuses on changing the client's current behavior. Efforts to change the client's behavior will be most effective when transfer of training is built into the treatment and the client is required to use new skills in multiple environments and conduct an ongoing self-evaluation of changes.

As mentioned at the beginning of this section, the intention was to provide a general strategy for treating the neurologically impaired juvenile sex offender. Given the difficulty of treating this client, it is recognized that many clinicians would feel uncomfortable if all that was available to guide treatment was a general strategy. It is necessary to have specific guidelines that can direct the clinicians' efforts as they interact with clients.

SPECIFIC GUIDELINES

Intervening with the neurologically impaired juvenile sex offender is largely determined by the nature of the client's disability. That is, the therapist should use interventions that circumvent or minimize the effects of the client's deficits. In this section, some of the more common neurological deficits will be discussed. In discussing these deficits, the nature of the impairment will be defined. Then, specific interventions designed to circumvent these impairments are presented. Finally, a clinical vignette is presented that illustrates both the nature of the disability and the method for circumventing the disability.

Attention

A good metaphor for understanding attention is to view it like a flashlight. In the dark, the only thing that a person can see is the thing struck by the beam of light from the flashlight. Attention is similar. Of all the buzzing and whirling activity in the environment, the thing that a person notices is the thing that receives the person's attention. If a person focuses his/her attention on relevant events or activities, then the person can maintain involvement in ongoing events. If a person's attention is focused on irrelevant activity, the person can appear detached, uninterested, or uninvolved. This is precisely the problem that is encountered when working with neurologically impaired juvenile sex offenders.

A survey of juvenile sex offenders in one program revealed that approximately 7 percent could be diagnosed with attention deficit disorder (ADD) and as many as 35 percent of the sample had some symptoms associated with this diagnosis (Kavoussi et al. 1988). As documented in the literature, the core problem associated with ADD is focusing and changing attention (Goldberg 1991). The prevalence of ADD among neurologically impaired sex offenders is unknown but it is expected to be commonplace. Therefore, the clinician must create an environment that minimizes the deleterious impact of the clients' attention problems.

Three techniques appear to be useful when contending with attention problems: (1) create a sparse environment, (2) provide parallel activities, and (3) use verbal and visual attention getters. These techniques are largely a matter of manipulating the client's environment, such that the client can focus on treatment. These techniques cannot always be done spontaneously. Some preparatory work may need to occur prior to meeting with the client.

A sparse environment is not necessarily an impoverished environment. A sparse environment is an environment in which the client will find few opportunities to engage in irrelevant or distracting behaviors. A sparse environment is characterized by a room with few objects that could be picked up or handled by clients. Ideally, furniture should be heavy so that clients cannot rock back or move the furniture. The treatment room should be large enough that clients cannot easily touch each other. Finally, the walls should be relatively free from distracting art or posters.

Once a sparse environment conducive to treatment has been created, the clients' ability and need to attend to multiple stimuli can be further molded. Clients with attention problems can use their distractibility as a strength by engaging in parallel therapeutic activities while other clients engage in verbal activities. For example, while one client talks about his offense, another client can be asked to write down any questions he wants to ask when the client is done. Another parallel activity would be to let one client use clay to sculpt his perception of the victim's face during the abuse that another group member is describing. The tactile, visual, and other sensory stimulation from the clay focuses the client's attention but the client is able to attend and remain involved in the verbal process. By engaging in a parallel yet related therapeutic activity the client's ability to attend to multiple stimuli is used constructively. Without such a parallel activity, the client might engage in side conversations or other distracting behaviors.

The third technique that has been effective in shaping a client's focus in a group is the use of attention getters. There are two types of attention getters: visual and verbal. Visual attention getters include posters, props, and other physical objects that are suddenly introduced during a therapy session. The visual attention getter should be used to direct attention or reinforce a new concept. Imagine the response of a client with an attention disorder when a child safety gate is brought out of a box and placed in a doorway as the clinician uses this prop to discuss self-control. The client's attention will probably be drawn from the other more predictable parts of the room to focus on this object. The novelty of this object will keep the client's attention focused on the discussion.

The other type of attention getter is the verbal attention getter. Consider the illustration below, in which a group of clients has little motivation to confront an unpopular new peer's thinking error:

New client: This is all that happened. The little boy that I was baby-sitting just came in the living room when my body was feeling horny. So, my body just made me have sex with him.

Clinician: Thanks, Johnny. Is there anything else you want to add?

New client: No, that is all that happened.

Clinician: Does anyone in the group want to ask Johnny about one thing he might have left out of his offense? (No response from peers.)

Clinician: (with excited voice tone) James, did you see what just happened here?

James: What do you mean?

Clinician: You didn't catch it? Hey, Bob, you have sort of been the group leader in the past. Tell the group what Johnny just did.

Bob: He just told what he did to his victim.

Clinician: (Turning his body back to face Johnny and lowering his voice somewhat.) Wow, Johnny, you are amazing. You just came to group and already you are more powerful than the group members who have been here for two or three months. They are letting you lead the group.

Bob: Johnny is not a group leader.

Clinician: Sure he is. The way Johnny used his power today was by negatively using several thinking errors, like "Feel It, Do It" and "Poor Me." Johnny was able to fool everyone because nobody else used his power by catching him and pointing out his thinking errors. The use of thinking errors always leads to negative feelings and acting-out behaviors. For that reason, I am wondering if we need to stop the group and relearn the thinking errors.

Verbal attention getters are always verbal interruptions of the group process. To the extent possible, the verbal attention getter should be startling but it cannot be too intense. If the counselor is too intense, it may stir up strong, primitive emotions among the clients. This could only serve to disorganize the clients, and consequently it would be difficult for them to focus attention.

Overall, the clinician can expect that the neurologically impaired juvenile sex offender will have attention problems. Since it is known that clients will have these problems, it would be prudent to anticipate and prepare for them. Due to the environmental manipulations that must occur, the clinician who wants to diminish the impact of attention problems must spend a great deal of time outside treatment preparing the environment.

Memory

One of the more frequently encountered symptoms in neurologically impaired persons is poor memory. It can be expected that many neurologically impaired sex offenders will have diminished memory capabilities. Still, it is important to realize that no client's memory impairment will be so severe that he has no memory at all. Clients will likely have sufficient memory to make them a risk for future acting out; they will have sufficient recall of their past deviance such that they could re-offend, if they choose to do so. It is this rudimentary memory that will also be used in treatment to help clients learn and use new skills designed to replace offense behavior.

The two techniques that seem most effective in diminishing the obstacles associated with poor memory are sequencing and redundancy. *Sequencing* refers to breaking down a complex skill or concept into the component parts and teaching the client on a piecemeal basis. Those in the behaviorist tradition will recognize this technique as successive approximation. The reason that this technique is effective is that clients find it easier to learn and recall information in small chunks, whereas recall of a complex skill or concept may be overwhelming. *Redundancy* refers to presenting information on multiple occasions. It is also useful to present information in different mediums, for example, visual, verbal, or kinesthetic. It is known that redundancy will keep information in short-term memory. It is also known that the longer information is maintained in short-term memory, the more likely it is to be transferred to long-term memory (Norman 1976).

In this clinical vignette of sequencing and redundancy, notice how the clinician weaves together these two techniques to make a powerful intervention with an entire group:

> *Johnny:* Hey, idiot, quit kicking my chair before I make you quit.
> *Clinician:* Johnny, stop. You need to do two things right now. One, you need to stop threatening. Two, you need to move your chair away from James's chair. Group, Johnny just tried to solve a problem. Did he solve it without getting into his cycle of abusive behavior?

Group members: No. Threatening is verbal abuse.

Clinician: That's right. Johnny, you did try to use the first step of the problem-solving process. The first step is to talk about the behavior that is a problem. You mentioned that James was kicking your chair. That is the problem behavior. Now, the second step is to say why that behavior is a problem. Johnny, can you try that again by putting step one and two together. Tell James what is the problem and *why* it is a problem.

Johnny: Well, I want you to stop touching my chair because it distracts me.

Clinician: That's right, you used the first and the second step of the problem-solving process. Bob, what process are we talking about?

Bob: The problem-solving process.

Clinician: That's right. James, what are the two steps of the problem-solving process that Johnny has already shown us?

James: Tell what's the problem and why.

Clinician: That's right. Pat yourself on the back. Now, Johnny, the last step, step three after telling what's the problem and why it's a problem is to tell what you can do about the problem. You threatened to make him stop without asking him to stop himself first. He might stop on his own, which would save the energy you might spend trying to make him stop. How can you tell James what you want done about the problem and save your energy?

Johnny: I can ask him to quit or tell him I'll switch chairs with someone else.

Clinician: Those are two good options. Now, tell James about the problem again using his name to get his attention. Use all three steps of the problem-solving process: state the problem, why it is a problem, and what you can do to solve it without abuse.

Johnny: OK. James, I don't like it when you are kicking my chair because it distracts me. I want you to stop and move your chair.

The foregoing illustrates how sequencing can be used to teach the client how to solve a problem using a problem that emerges during a therapy session. In addition to sequencing, repetition was also used. The steps in the sequence were repeated several times by the clinician and by the clients who were drawn into the process. As the clinician spoke about each step, he/she could have held up one, two, or three fingers to indicate the step in the process. This visual cue might enhance memory for someone with deficits in verbal memory but strengths in visual memory. A small chart with three icons depicting the three steps in the problem-solving process could also be used as a visual cue. Communicating the same concept in different mediums is a form of redundancy.

Memory impairment may be the ultimate determinant of how quickly and how far a client will progress. The more severe the memory impairment, the slower the progress and the more guarded the prognosis. Clinicians must develop appropriate expectations for progress on a client-by-client basis, and memory may be the most critical factor in formulating these expectations.

Language Disorders

There are two types of language disorders: expressive and receptive. An expressive language disorder is characterized by a person's inability to put ideas, concepts, or feelings into words. It is not that a person does not have knowledge. In an expressive language disorder the person does have the knowledge but cannot find the words. In many ways, the expressive language disorder is similar to the tip-of-the-tongue phenomenon, that is, you know a word but it eludes your recall. As might be expected, expressive language problems can be very frustrating.

A receptive language problem occurs when a person cannot encode and decode speech in a reliable manner. That is, the person with a receptive language disorder fails to understand what is being said. This deficit, also, is not due to a lack of knowledge. Oftentimes the person with a receptive language disorder knows and uses the very words or sentences that he/she cannot comprehend when others speak. A good way to understand the receptive language disorder is that it is a form of dyslexia for the ears.

The client with an expressive language problem could be expected to have difficulty verbalizing thoughts or responding to questions. He might use short sentences, give tangential responses, omit critical parts of sentences, or substitute incorrect words in sentences. He often has difficulty learning new words or recalling new words. It is important for the clinician to distinguish between circumventions, or roundabout speech, due to expressive language deficits, and defensiveness, in which the client is purposely attempting to evade answering a question directly. Since the ability to be direct is impaired with a language disorder, the client requires verbal modeling. Deficits in language should not be viewed as defensiveness might be. The correct response to a deficit is to teach or compensate.

The client with receptive language impairments may have multiple problems with areas of auditory processing (e.g., encoding, storage, and recall) or understanding complex and abstract statements. It is important for the clinician to distinguish between resistance and impaired receptive language. The proper response to resistance is a confrontation. The proper response to impaired receptive language is to help the client input verbal information. For example, the clinician can ask the client to repeat his understanding of the question to determine if the client has adequately understood a verbal interaction. Most clients will try to hide their deficits. The clinician should routinely ascertain the client's understanding of the verbal interaction.

Three techniques are useful when treating clients with language disorders: (1) *maximum auditory stimulation* — new words or concepts are repeated several times and explained several different ways (Tompkins 1991); (2) *multisensory cues* — the same information is presented through different sensory media; and (3) *verbal modeling* — an example and an opportunity are provided for the client to practice verbalizations. In the vignette that follows, notice how the clinician used all three techniques simultaneously to create a powerful intervention with a group of clients:

Clinician: Today we are going to learn how to use covert sensitization to change urges for deviant sex. Covert sensitization is a big name for a simple process. Covert sensitization has three parts. The first two parts of covert sensitization are negative, like sitting in a hot seat. The third part of covert sensitization is like a peaceful recliner where most people can enjoy life for awhile. Johnny, these three chairs represent the covert sensitization process. What do the chairs stand for?

Johnny: Covert sensitization.

Clinician: That's right. James, two chairs or two parts of covert sensitization are negative like hot seats. Which parts or chairs are the negative ones?

James: The closest ones.

Clinician: OK. The closest ones are which chairs?

James: Oh, the first and second chairs are the hot seats chairs.

Clinician: Right. Now, Bob, would you come up here and give us an example of each step by sitting in each chair? I am going to put a cutout of flames on the first two seats to remind everyone that these seats get hot if you stay too long. I am going to put a pillow on the third chair to remind everyone that the third chair or third step is where you want to spend most of your time to change a deviant urge. . . . (The explanations continue with details of the covert sensitization process: recognizing the urge and stopping before thinking of the actual deviant sex; thinking of real consequences to self and other if deviant sex occurred, while stopping before dwelling on pain to self and other; and spending time thinking of acting on choices for alternative pro-social behaviors that can leave one feeling good for a long time.)

The clinician in the foregoing example helped the clients with receptive language disorder by repeating the term *covert sensitization* many times. The chairs, flames, and pillow act as multisensory cues to help the process of storing and sequencing the information about covert sensitization. The chairs, flames, and pillow also provide visual cues as they are pointed to when each step is discussed. The chairs provide auditory cues as each one is moved forward as that step is discussed. As individuals take turns sitting in the chairs and reciting personal examples of each step, the tactile sensation of moving quickly from the first two chairs and relaxing in the third chair helps each individual recall which step to spend the most time on. To help clients with an expressive language disorder, note that the clinician helped the clients communicate by asking simple fill-in-the-blank questions. The clinician also helped a client elaborate on a simple answer.

Perhaps the best way to conceptualize the clinician's role with regard to language deficits is that the clinician fills in the gaps. When dealing with clients with expressive language disorders, the clinician helps the client find the missing word. When dealing with receptive language disorders, the clinician assists by providing multiple-input options, and hopefully, one input will assist the client in comprehending. Overall, the clinician cannot assume that the client can express or comprehend. Rather, the clinician must be prepared to help clients with each of these tasks.

Reading Disorders

Juvenile sex offenders are sometimes referred to as the "hidden offenders" because they appear average in academic achievement when compared to other youths (Milloy 1994). However, there is nothing about the academic achievement of the neurologically impaired juvenile sex offender that would result in him being "hidden." To the contrary, the neurologically impaired juvenile sex offender, like other neurologically impaired youths, tends to do poorly in school.

Reading deficits are often the most common of the academic problems exhibited by the neurologically impaired juvenile sex offender.

Reading disorders result in problems during the assessment phase and throughout treatment. During the assessment, it may be the intention of the clinician to assess the client by use of paper and pencil tests. However, most paper and pencil tests require that a person be able to read at the sixth- or eighth-grade level. Many neurologically impaired juvenile sex offenders are capable of no more than a third- or forth-grade reading level. Once the client makes it past the assessment and begins treatment, the reading deficit may be even more debilitating. Most sex offender treatment programs require that the client read assignments and worksheets. Progress depends upon the client's ability to respond to written materials. Progress is slow or nonexistent when the client lacks the requisite reading skills.

Somehow the clinician must find a way to circumvent the problems caused by a client's poor reading skills. In principle, this is accomplished by replacing written assignments with auditory or nonverbal visual substitutes. Two techniques seem to be particularly useful when contending with reading disorders: (1) *visual nonverbal material*—to the extent possible, written material should be recoded to a pictorial representation, for example, the use of icons to represent thinking errors; and (2) *auditory presentations*—put standard tests, assignments, and lectures on audiotape so that clients can listen rather than read. Both of these techniques should be used when a client is suspected of having a reading disorder.

Brain Irritability

A common feature of neurologically impaired behavior is its unmodulated, extreme presentation. Emotions tend to be expressed in their raw, primitive form. There is little modulation or sublimation of intense motives. In general, the neurologically impaired person appears agitated and aggressive. Among neurologically impaired juvenile sex offenders impulse control disorder and explosive disorders are common. Many neurologically impaired juvenile sex offenders have multiple episodes of impulsive or aggressive acting out. Sometimes this behavior is associated with a catastrophic reaction, that is, the client acts out in response to being disabled (Goldstein 1952). At other times, the juvenile sex offender may merely be acting in accordance with his own deviant or antisocial motives. Regardless of the cause, aggressive acting out should be recognized as countertherapeutic, and to the extent possible it should be curtailed. Two techniques seem to be useful when trying to curtail aggressive outbursts: scaffolding and relaxation techniques.

Scaffolding is a term that refers to providing a framework or foundation for other group processes. In group therapy, the group rules, contracts, orientation sessions, stages of treatment, and layout format provide scaffolding. A client who has simple, concrete rituals and structures like these has less reason to feel frustrated or irritable in a therapy session. The scaffolding provides consistency and predictability, which decrease the amount of tension a client might experience.

Relaxation techniques are also effective with aggressive youth. Relaxation techniques need to be taught to the client prior to the time that he needs to use them. Clients should be taught to use the techniques whenever tension begins to build. Some types of relaxation techniques include guided visualizations at the beginning or end of group sessions, deep breathing exercises, paced breathing exercises, progressive muscle relaxation, and relaxation audiotapes. A creative approach to relaxation training is to have group members create a five-minute relaxation tape. Then, at the beginning of the group session, a client may play his relaxation tape.

Another idea is to let each client choose his own type of relaxation music or visualization to put on his tape. The tapes are something the client can take from treatment to use in the community.

Brain irritability is largely a matter of a low threshold for frustration tolerance. Clients will have good days and bad days with regard to brain irritability but one thing is certain: there will be bad days. It is too late to start dealing with brain irritability once the client begins to act out. As in other forms of aggression control, the clinician must be proactive and prevent acting out episodes by use of scaffolding. When scaffolding fails, as it will from time to time, it is important to have already taught clients how to engage in self-regulation through the use of relaxation techniques.

CONCLUSIONS

The neurologically impaired juvenile sex offender presents a unique clinical picture. Consequently, many standard therapy techniques cannot be utilized unless these techniques are modified to match the unique characteristics of these clients. In this chapter, a general strategy was suggested for working with the neurologically impaired juvenile sex offender. It was suggested that these clients be viewed as similar to severe character disorders or primitive personalities. Much has been written in the past thirty years regarding effective strategies for intervening with this type of disorder. The clinician who chooses to work with the neurologically impaired juvenile sex offender is encouraged to follow the strategy articulated in this literature, that is, focus on existing behavior and strive to increase the client's self-control. In the process of attempting to intervene with the neurologically impaired juvenile sex offender it is recognized that a general strategy is necessary but not sufficient. That is why most of this chapter was devoted to discussing issues of learning, attention, memory, language, reading problems, and impulsivity. These issues are often the most problematic for the clinician as the client's deficits in these areas often serve to impede or disrupt therapy. While it is possible to formulate interventions that can circumvent the debilitating effect of these disabilities, one thing should remain obvious: therapy with the neurologically impaired juvenile sex offender is possible but progress will be slow and success will depend upon the clinician's ability to minimize the effect of the client's deficits.

4

The Bridges Program

Successful treatment of the neurologically impaired juvenile sex offender depends largely upon the clinician's ability to circumvent or minimize the interference caused by the client's neurological impairments. This type of treatment puts quite a burden upon the clinician. The clinician must do more than just guide the client. The clinician must also build the road so that the client may progress on the therapeutic journey. Perhaps the most important role played by the therapist is to provide a bridge from one of the client's areas of functioning to another area of functioning. In providing this bridge, the clinician circumvents the client's deficits in functioning.

Parmeley (1994) provides a visual representation of treatment with neurologically impaired clients. She suggests that treatment is like driving a vehicle from one town to another. Imagine that the car in Figure 4–1 is a neurologically impaired juvenile sex offender who is seeking treatment. The roads on the map are therapeutic avenues that the client must travel to reach the treatment goal. The neurological impairment is like an earthquake that leaves fissures in the path the client must follow. For the client to succeed, bridges must be built to span the gaps in the roads. Since the program developed is based upon the notion that the clinician must build bridges if the client is to progress, this treatment program for the neurologically impaired juvenile sex offender is called the Bridges Program.

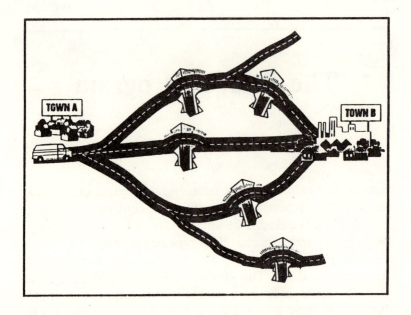

Figure 4–1.

BASIC CONCEPTS

The National Task Force of Juvenile Sex Offender Treatment (National Council of Juvenile and Family Court Judges
1993) provides guidelines for those who work with juvenile
sex offenders. The comprehensive list of therapeutic activities recommended by the National Task Force was used to
create the Bridges Program. Six key issues serve as the
program's foundation:

Positive sexuality—Youths who enter the program typically have little awareness of positive sexual attitudes or
behaviors. The sexual attitudes and information they
possess promote deviant sexual behavior. Consequently,
one issue they must address is the development of positive
sexual attitudes and knowledge.

Offense cycle — The offense cycle is the youths' personal pattern of deviant sexual behavior. Youths are taught to recognize their own offense cycle so they can stop their cycle before it results in harm to others.

Victim empathy — Empathy is the ability to recognize, and even resonate with, the thoughts and feelings of another person. Ryan and Lane (1991) suggest that the desire for sexual intimacy and immediate gratification are at odds in sexual offending, that is, the offender uses sex instead of intimacy to feel good. Clients must come to recognize how their behavior has impact on others, especially those whom they have harmed. The purpose of increased empathy is to develop within the client a feeling that could prevent sexual misconduct.

Restitution — The victims of sex offenses never deserved to be harmed. To the contrary, they deserve to be given back those things that the offender took as a result of the offense. Restitution involves restoring, or giving back, some of the things that were harmed as a result of the sexual offense. Emotional restitution is the goal that an offender should endeavor to achieve. The offender should strive to restore the victim's positive emotional state that existed prior to the victimization.

Relapse prevention — It is easy to quit engaging in a problematic behavior. The difficulty occurs when the person tries to stay quit. Many clients can learn to change their attitudes and behaviors; however, success depends upon maintaining these changes. Relapse prevention refers to the activities designed to help the client hold onto positive new behavior and prevent reverting back to negative behavior.

Thinking errors — A person's beliefs determine his/her view of the world. Beliefs also influence behavior. The beliefs held by juvenile sex offenders promote deviant sexual behavior. Yochelson and Samenow (1976) have identified very specific beliefs held by sex offenders. A client's success in treatment is largely determined by the client's ability to recognize and eliminate criminal thinking patterns.

These six issues are the focus of treatment in the Bridges Program. Other issues could be addressed in treatment, but when treating clients with neurological deficits, it is important to do a few things well rather than overextend. Even though the scope of the Bridges Program is limited, the issues addressed in the program are core issues that must be addressed with neurologically impaired clients. That is the essence of specialized treatment—the economical use of specific interventions for a specific problem.

STAGES OF TREATMENT

There are five stages of treatment in the Bridges Program: one orientation stage and four treatment stages. During the orientation stage, the client learns how to succeed in treatment. During the treatment stages, the six therapeutic issues are addressed in a variety of ways, depending on the stage of treatment. Consider the main theme and purpose of each treatment stage:

Stage One: Concept Formation—The client is introduced to the six basic issues that compose the treatment program.
Stage Two: Transfer of Training—The client is assigned tasks that require him to address the six issues in settings other than therapy.
Stage Three: Generalization and Practice—The client continues to develop coping skills and he is required to use these skills in all areas of his life.

Stage Four: Transition Planning—The client begins making plans and contacting key persons who will be involved in his aftercare.

The Bridges Program can be reduced to a matrix (Table 4–1). Along the rows, the six therapeutic issues are listed. The columns are labeled according to the stages of treatment. In creating such a matrix, it becomes clear that redundancy and multiple context training are incorporated into the program design.

Clients who suffer from neurological impairments will benefit from the redundancy built into the Bridges Program. Much effort was devoted to ensuring that therapeutic tasks do not rely primarily upon the client's verbal skills. Notice that clients are asked to develop games, write songs, engage in role play, and make posters. Most of these tasks entail visual or interpersonal skills, not verbal skills. It was hoped that by using these interventions, it would be possible to circumvent, or bridge, the deficits caused by the client's neurological impairments.

Having introduced the notion that each of the six therapeutic issues is dealt with repeatedly throughout treatment, we now further delineate these tasks. All therapeutic tasks in the program can be found in the Bridges Program Client

Table 4–1.
Matrix of Treatment

Stages and Treatment Issues	*Stages of Treatment*			
	One	*Two*	*Three*	*Four*
Healthy sexuality	Pictures	Book report	Role play	Plan
Offense cycle	Poster	Game	Lesson plan	Plan
Victim empathy	Role play	Homework	Card game	Plan
Victim restitution	Letter	Role play	Letter	Plan
Relapse prevention	Worksheet	Song	Plan	Schedule
Thinking errors	Worksheet	Homework	Poster	Plan

Workbook (see Appendix A). An explanation and instructions for each task in the workbook are presented. Tasks are grouped according to their place in the client workbook. The binding agreements, the orientation process, and the tasks comprising the four treatment stages are discussed.

Binding Agreements

Topic: Stages of treatment
Purpose: To provide clients with guidelines and markers of their progress through treatment.
Description: The stages of treatment contain a listing of all therapeutic tasks and goals that a client must achieve in order to complete the program.
Directions: 1. Read through the stages of treatment with the client and answer any general questions about the stages.
               2. Advise the clients that they must complete all stages of treatment in order to graduate from this program.
               3. Point out that additional tasks may be required if the client completes all other tasks before completing the goals of each stage.
               4. Explain that staff will sign off on each task or goal as soon as it is completed. Clarify that the clients may not sign and date when tasks are completed.
Topic: Treatment contract
Purpose: To educate and hold the client accountable for safe, nonabusive behavior while at the facility.
Description: The treatment contract includes guidelines for interacting with victims and potential victims, control of deviant outlets, therapeutic activities, and confidentiality. The treatment con-

tract is signed by the client and the clinician when the client understands and agrees to follow these guidelines between and within group sessions.

Directions: 1. Give the client a copy of the contract to read. If the client cannot read, the clinician can read it to him. Clients with receptive language disorders and borderline intellectual functioning are asked to repeat their understanding of each statement to assure they correctly understand each guideline. The clinician can help the clients understand items by describing situations where the client would have to apply that guideline.

2. Clients are asked to circle any guideline they don't understand or can't agree with.

3. After the other guidelines are covered, the clinician can return to circled guidelines to further explore each one with the client.

4. Any client who does not agree to all items must not sign the contract. The clinician can use collateral sources to help resistant clients understand the importance of each guideline. For example, if a client insists upon talking to a younger incest victim on the phone because he feels it would upset the victim if he did not have such contact, the clinician can talk to the offender's parents to secure support for the client to not have contact with the young victim.

5. The client signs the contract once he agrees to abide by it. The clinician who explained the treatment contract to the client signs also.

6. The treatment contract is kept in the client's file.

Topic: Group rules contract

Purpose: To educate and contract with the client to follow rules that enhance group functioning.

Description: The group rules were created by former clients of the Bridges Program. These rules address hygiene, basic interactions skills, and client responsibilities. When a client signs these rules before entering group, the client has made a commitment to behave in a manner that promotes therapeutic progress. In essence, the group rules are a prescription for succeeding in group therapy.

Directions: 1. The client is given a copy of the group rules to read. The client circles any items he does not understand or support. If a client cannot read or has a receptive language disorder, the clinician should read each item and ask the client to repeat his understanding of each item.

              2. The clients should be asked to pick one or two items that they feel they may have problems with. Clients should be requested to develop a specific plan of dealing with these problem areas.

Prestage: Orientation

There are two therapeutic tasks in this stage: truth worksheet and orientation quiz. It should be noted, however, that much of the orientation is accomplished by reviewing with the client the information contained in the orientation section of the client workbook. The clinician is encouraged to use the material in this section of the client workbook to teach the client about therapy. The clinician should review with the client the material in the orientation section and ensure that the client understands this material.

Topic: Truth worksheet
Purpose: To begin the disclosure with staff, group members, and family.
Description: The first order of business when dealing with a sex offender is to get the offender to admit to a problem with deviant sex. The client needs to minimize denial and increase accountability. Since most persons who use deviant sex do not readily or openly discuss their sexuality, the Bridges Program allows the client to reveal himself through a worksheet. The truth worksheet helps the client begin to recognize and admit to using deviant sexual behavior. The manner in which the client completes the worksheet may reveal the amount of sexual knowledge and empathy the client brings to group.
Directions: 1. The clinician gives a copy of the truth worksheet to the client. If the client cannot write or has an expressive language disorder, the clinician can accept the client's dictation and/or help the client with each question.

2. When this is done, the clinician and client need to discuss the client's answers to assess the client's level of self-knowledge, victim empathy, and awareness of grooming patterns. It is important for the client and clinician to begin identifying the issues that the client must address to avoid re-offending.

3. The clinician should arrange for the client to be on the agenda of the next treatment team meeting. During this meeting, the client is given the opportunity to present the truth worksheet. It is the clinician's job to ensure that the client leaves the treatment team

meeting feeling supported by and accountable to all treatment team members.

4. The clinician confers with the client's family therapist to secure a time slot during the next family therapy session for the client to present the truth worksheet to family members. Ideally, the family needs to discuss how they can support the client in treatment. The clinician should be available during this portion of family therapy. To the extent possible, the clinician should attempt to help the family decrease denial and deal with the pain associated with accepting that the client has displayed deviant sex. The clinician needs to support parents who raise questions or appear distressed.

5. When all other orientation work is complete, the clinician arranges for the client to enter a sex offender group therapy session. The client is permitted to present his/her truth worksheet during the first group therapy session.

Topic: Orientation quiz

Purpose: To provide clients an opportunity to review what they learned in the orientation program.

Description: Because of the large amount of material that was introduced to the client during orientation, it is important to assess the client's understanding and ability to retain the information presented. If the client shows some difficulty learning the information, it may help to review specific orientation materials. If this does not help the client pass the quiz on the second administration, it may indicate a need to revise teaching strategies.

Directions: 1. If the client can read well, let the client read and answer questions on the quiz. Otherwise, dictate the quiz and record the client's answers.
2. If the client incorrectly answers any of the first four questions, ask the client to look through the packet of materials and review the handout or worksheet that addresses the questions.
3. Praise the client who searches for answers. Also, praise the client who does not act out when he/she does not have correct answers the first time.
4. Sign and date this line of the stages of treatment form when the quiz has been filled in correctly by the client.

Stage One: Concept Formation

Tasks in this stage are designed to teach the client new skills for self-control.

Topic: Layout
Purpose: To remind clients of why they are in the group, of their responsibility to follow the treatment contract, and of their responsibility to have a topic each week to discuss. It is also designed to increase accountability and self-monitoring of deviant urges and other behaviors related to the client's sexual abuse cycle.
Description: During each group session a client has the opportunity to regress into denial or to fantasize about deviant sex. For these reasons, each session is very structured.

At the beginning of each group therapy

session, the client should recite his layout. Each part of the layout was designed for a specific purpose. The first line asks for the client's name. This is important as the clients often depersonalize others by saying "that guy," "that girl," or "what's-his-name over there." The second line asks what offense(s) brought the client to group. This was designed to decrease the client's denial about why they are in group. The acceptable answers here include "sexual abuse," "rape," "molestation," "sexual assault," or "peeping." Unacceptable answers that indicate minimization include "doing something to a little boy" or "hurting my stepsister." The third line asks the client to identify all victims by name. When a victim's name is not known, the client may be instructed to describe the victim's age and give a name, e.g., "A 6-year-old girl I will call Jane." Again, the purpose is to keep clients from depersonalizing others, especially victims. The fourth line asks the client to list all other abusive power-based behaviors that support the cycle of abuse, even when there is no opportunity for the client to sexually abuse others. This line is for accountability and may be amplified as the client gains more sophisticated self-awareness.

The fifth line of the layout is a reminder that all clients in the Bridges Program have a responsibility to follow the treatment contract. This line increases self-awareness and self-monitoring of how well they know and follow the guidelines. Peers may be asked to confront the client on any unreported or suspected infractions to increase honesty and accountability to the group. The sixth line asks the clients to estimate how many impulses for deviant sex or abusive behavior the client experienced since the last group session. The clients are then asked to list what positive coping resources were used. It is important not to allow clients to discuss details of their deviant or abusive impulses. If the group is aware that the client acted out aggressively or abusively and the client does not report these behaviors, the client's peers are expected to report the behavior. The last line asks the client to state the topic he needs to discuss during that group session. The topic should relate to the tasks and goals as listed in the stage of treatment. If the client brings up a concern, the clinician can ask the client which tool in the current stage of treatment might apply to the current problem. It is acceptable for the client to use group to discuss perpetration issues or progress in family therapy sessions in which perpetration issues are discussed.

Directions: 1. The client can find the layout sheet in the client workbook.
2. In the first group, the client writes answers on the initial layout form as group members describe the purpose of each line.
3. In subsequent groups, clients complete layouts verbally, making written additions as they gain self-awareness.
4. Clients assertively determine the order of presenting the layouts to practice sharing time and leadership.
5. Clients are told they are responsible for knowing basic information in peers' layouts so they may take notes if necessary. These

notes must be kept in their folders.

6. After topics are given, one member may be asked to keep a list of them. Then members are asked to prioritize issues and split group time.

Topic: Positive sex versus deviant sex

Purpose: To begin educating clients on the difference between positive and deviant sex.

Description: Most sex offenders have distorted ideas about sex due to their own sexual abuse, premature exposure to adult sexual behaviors, or exposure to deviant sex in sexually explicit media. The purpose of this worksheet is to provide concrete criteria for clients to memorize and apply to sexual urges and behaviors. Then, the clients may begin to distinguish between healthy sex and deviant sex.

Directions: 1. Have the client read the healthy vs. deviant sex worksheet in a group therapy session. The client is instructed to give a personal example for each of the criteria of positive and deviant sex. Have the clients use actual examples from their own sexual history to show they understand each characteristic.

2. Have the client pass the paper to a neighbor and repeat the criteria to show they memorized them.

3. In a subsequent group therapy session, have the client's peers quiz him on the criteria.

4. Encourage the client to use and refer to these criteria when discussing healthy and deviant aspects of sexual behaviors and urges.

Topic: Offense cycle poster

Purpose: To help clients uncover and control their personal pattern of deviant sexual behavior.

Description: Each client has his/her own pattern of behaviors that precede deviant sex. Since many neurologically impaired clients may have trouble controlling their impulses and understanding sequences of events, they may believe deviant sex just happens. Experience has shown that these offenders sometimes feel powerless over stopping their deviant sexual behaviors since they are faced with limitations in other areas of functioning also. Most juveniles quickly comprehend the offense cycle when it is presented to them. Learning about the offense cycle can be uplifting to neurologically impaired clients as they begin to develop self-awareness. Ultimately clients use their self-awareness to interrupt the pattern and stop deviant sexual behavior. The cycle follows these five steps in order:

Stressful Event — A stressful event is any unpleasant interaction or situation, such as arguments with peers, being teased due to learning problems, or not being able to remember something they were just told.

Negative Self-Talk — Self-talk is what a person says silently. It is what the person thinks about. People who practice deviant sex have many negative thoughts in their self-talk. These thoughts usually include thinking errors (Yochelson and Samenow 1976).

Fantasy — A fantasy is a visual representation of how we would like things to be. Deviant sexual fantasies usually provide strong arousal. Fantasy keeps the person motivated. Some people masturbate while having a deviant sex fantasy to increase the pleasure associated with the fantasy.

Grooming—This is the interaction between the offender and the victim in which the offender isolates and sets up the victim. The victim is usually unaware of being groomed.

Deviant Sex—This is sex that hurts the victim.

Because of their short-term memory deficits and rigid thinking patterns, juvenile sex offenders with neurological impairment may believe they have stopped their cycle whenever a short period of time elapses since they last engaged in deviant sex. This is why it is important to help each youth become aware of how this cycle leads to other unacceptable behaviors. The other unacceptable behavior usually involves feeling pleasure by having power over someone else in a way that hurts others (e.g., provoking, lying, stealing, intimidating, physically assaulting, etc.).

Directions: 1. Show the client the offense cycle poster with the five steps and symbols on it. Give the client the offense cycle handout. Have the client cut out five pieces and put them on the table in a circle in order. The client can point to each piece of paper as he answers the following questions:

   A. *Deviant sex*—What is a deviant sex act you committed? Who was the victim? When and where did it happen?

   B. *Grooming*—How did you get the victim to trust you? What did you do to gain access to the victim? How did you keep your plan a secret? How did you isolate the victim or get the victim alone?

   C. *Fantasy*—What were the pictures in your mind about this sex act? What did you want to do to the victim? How did you think the victim would react?

D. *Negative Self-Talk* — What thinking errors did you use regarding the stressful event? What thinking errors did you use when you began to plan the deviant sex act?

E. *Stressful Event* — Give the date, time, and place of the stressful event that triggered the offense cycle.

2. After working through the steps of the offense cycle during a group session, the client is given a homework assignment: The client uses a large sheet of poster paper and draws the cycle steps using one color of marker. Then using another color of marker, the client can list his personal steps of the cycle. Then the client presents his poster to group members during a group therapy session.

3. Have the client revise the offense cycle homework according to the feedback that the client receives from group members.

4. Have the client revise and present the offense cycle homework until it is approved by the group members, the group therapists, and the client's primary therapist.

Topic: Victim's story

Purpose: To help the client see the deviant sexual act from the victim's point of view.

Description: The neurologically impaired offender is very concrete in his/her thinking. If a victim smiled during the abuse, the offender may assume the victim enjoyed the abuse. If the victim said nothing, the offender might assume the victim was not emotionally affected by the abuse. Concrete thinkers do not consider a blank stare as a manifestation of confusion, terror, or shock. These offenders often do not have a large-enough fund of sexual information to understand that a body may respond to a pleasurable touch while responding emotionally in a negative way to the situation in which the pleasurable touch is occurring.

The goal of this exercise is to educate juvenile sex offenders about the true effects of their behavior on the victim. It is designed to help the offenders understand how they might misread social cues. It might further help the offenders understand the differences between their perception and the victim's perception.

Directions: 1. Have the client sit in a chair in the middle of the group. Let the client tell his/her victim's story about the abuse. Make sure the client describes the abuse from the victim's perspective and not his/her own. Remind the client to use the words the victim might use at that age. Remind the client to describe the victim's perception of events before, during, and after the abuse.

2. Have the other group members ask questions of the "victim" to help the client expand his/her understanding of the "victim's" perspective.

3. Have the client repeat this task for each victim.

4. Continue to revise the victim story until accepted by group members and clinician.

Topic: Clarification letter

Description: Victims deserve to hear the offender take responsibility and try to answer the question "why." But the clarification letter is also helpful to the offenders. By completing this task, the clients expand their understanding to include the fact that past deviant sexual behaviors are not part of the past until the offenders attempt to answer the questions victims may have about the past abuse. Ideally, the client should present the clarification letter to the victim. When this is not possible, the letter, or videotape, can be sent to the victim or victim's therapist to aid in the victim's healing.

Directions:

1. Give the client the clarification handout. Based upon the client's ability, have the client complete the form in writing or verbally.

2. During a group session, have the client read the letter filling in the blanks. Use group feedback to help the client make sure he/she is not blaming the victim or minimizing responsibility. Help the client use what he/she learned about the characteristics of healthy versus deviant sex and the offense cycle, when applicable. Again, redundancy is crucial to these clients. Make sure the client revises the letter using the feedback received during the group session.

3. When a letter receives group approval, it may be sent, or videotaped to send, to the victim's therapist. In cases where the victim desires no contact from the offender, the letter should be kept in the client's folder.

4. A client should complete a clarification letter for each victim. The clinician can provide feedback on subsequent letters or let the client read others to the group, depending on time constraints.

Topic: Stay away, look away, get away worksheet

Purpose: To allow the client to develop specific coping skills for dealing with high-risk situations.

Description: For the clients to break their cycle, they need to acquire coping skills. Furthermore, clients must learn to use these coping skills in situations that may result in sexual acting out. For the client to develop and use coping skills in these situations, the skills must be very simple and easy to remember. Clients can use the following three skills to cope with any situation that typically leads to sexual acting out and other forms of acting out:

Stay away—This skill requires that a person avoid or not go near persons or situations associated with urges for acting-out behaviors.

Look away—This skill requires that a client use a cognitive skill such as covert sensitization, punishment scenes, or aversive scenes. This is necessary when the situation precludes an avoiding or escaping response.

Get away—This coping skill entails escaping or leaving a high-risk situation. Clients are taught that some high-risk situations may come as a surprise or develop quickly. Still, the client must do something to cope.

Directions: 1. Give the client two worksheets to complete verbally or in writing. One should relate to the use of stay away, look away, get away as it pertains to behavior during treatment sessions. One should relate to use of these skills elsewhere at this facility.

2. The client must read and revise both sheets with feedback received from the group.

Topic: Positive attitude worksheets
Purpose: To help clients recognize and change distorted thinking patterns.
Description: See the handout on "Thinking Errors" in the orientation section of the client workbook.
Directions: 1. Give each client fourteen positive attitude worksheets.

2. During a group session, explain how the client should fill out each part.
   A. Name—client's name.
   B. Date the worksheet is filled out.
   C. Write about a problem behavior that occurred that day or draw about a problem behavior that occurred.
   D. Circle the smart self-talk icon that could have led to more adaptive behavior.
   E. Write or draw about three other situations that might prove that the smart self-talk is true.
3. Give the client an example using the thinking error "I can't" and smart self-talk "I can." Use a large sheet of paper to draw a sample copy of the worksheet. Let clients take turns filling in parts of the worksheet.
4. Let the clients fill out up to three worksheets per group, for a minimum of five sessions.

Stage Two: Transfer of Training

The purpose of this stage of treatment is to expand upon the concepts introduced in stage one. At this point in treatment, clients have begun to reduce their denial about deviant sex and increase their motivation for healthy sexual expression. All of the progress clients have made has occurred around staff and peers who are familiar with the treatment program. Unfortunately, deviant thoughts and urges do not occur exclusively while the client is in a special therapy group. Deviant impulses can occur anytime. Most of an adolescent's time is spent at school and around peers where seeking approval is the norm. This stage of treatment focuses on helping the client carry new concepts and skills into everyday situations, where deviant thoughts are most likely to occur. If the client cannot cope in different situations on campus, the client is less likely to be able to cope in the future. Therefore, this stage of treatment challenges the client to use skills in new situations.

Topic: Deviant sex versus healthy sex

Purpose: To provide an activity to increase the client's understanding and use of principles that distinguish healthy sex from deviant sex.

Description: Since the client was required previously to discuss healthy sex openly and confront characteristics of deviant sex within group discussions, it is time to broaden the use of these principles. In this task, the client has two options for owning and discussing his/her support of healthy sexual expression. One option is for the client to create a poster with pictures of attractive, interesting people that do not focus on anyone's sexual body parts. The other option is for a client to write a book report. By writing a book report, the client gains validation for his/her understanding of the principles of healthy sexuality from a source other than the client workbook.

Topic: Book report

Directions: 1. The clients choose an article from the clinician's library or from the school library on the topic of sexual behavior. This article must be approved by the clinician.

                2. The clients must take the article and book report form to their teacher and ask if they can receive school credit for this report. If so, the report can be written in class. If not, the report can be written during leisure time.

                3. After the client reads the article, the book report form should be completed. If the cli-

ent has difficulty writing, the book report may be audiotaped.

4. The book report is presented in a group therapy session and discussed.

5. Staff and peers attempt to determine if the client has a better understanding of healthy sex. Feedback is given to help the client further define the characteristics of healthy sex.

Topic: The cycle game

Purpose: To provide repetition of the steps and sequence in the offense cycle so that the client may increase self-control and self-awareness.

Description: The client must create a game based upon the offense cycle. Then, the client must teach the game to others during a group therapy session. Any type of game can be created. Action games such as basketball's P.I.G. game can be adapted to fit stages in the cycle. Card games or board games can be created. Other action games can be used such as charades or a picture game in which steps are acted out or drawn out for others to guess.

Directions:
1. The client is asked to think about a familiar word game, board game, card game, or action game that he can teach others.

2. Once the client selects a game, he must discuss his idea with peers during a group therapy session.

3. After the client decides on a game, materials can be requested from the clinician.

4. The client must explain and play the game with peers during a group therapy session.

5. Afterward, the client needs to process how it felt to teach something new to others. The client can be asked to consider how it might feel to express new thoughts about breaking

the cycle around peers who support deviant sex. The group members need to help the client explore how he can get help from friends to break the cycle while revealing a great deal or just a little about this issue.

Topic: Empathy homework

Purpose: To provide a structured task to help the client transfer the value of showing empathy to a larger population.

Description: In stage one the client learned to consider how his behavior hurts another. The simple message of that activity is that it is not okay to hurt others. Although clients may acquire an awareness of empathy, it is important that they practice being empathic.

Directions: 1. At least once a day, for one week, the client must encourage peers to consider how their actions might affect others and encourage them to avoid harmful behaviors.

                2. The client must have a staff member initial the goal card one time for seven days when the client is observed doing this.

                3. At the end of a week the client turns in the goal card and discusses his experiences. The client may be asked: Did people notice a difference in your attitude? Did they believe what you were saying? Did you care about the people you asked your peers not to harm? How would you feel doing this consistently around others?

Topic: "The Gifts" exercise

Purpose: To provide an opportunity for repetition of the concept of restitution for hurtful behavior.

Description: This task builds on the stage one task, the clarification letter. Like that task, the gifts exercise guides the client to consider how victims are harmed and how they suffer. The gifts exercise encourages the clients to focus on what they have in common with other people. Throughout this task, clients explore how those with good self-esteem see the good in others and how self-esteem plays a role in valuing others.

Directions:

1. Have the client select a peer to help with role play. Provide props such as gift-wrapped boxes. The client is "the teen."

2. The clinician will read "The Gifts" story a few lines at a time while the client role plays the story.

3. Have the client take three "gifts" worksheets. On each, have the client choose one staff member or peer he/she recently mistreated in some way.

4. Have the client put that person's name on the bottom line.

5. Then have the client write across the person's shoes one bad thing about the person that the client used to justify acting out toward that person.

6. Then have the client write or draw symbols in each "gift" box for one good quality that person possesses, which the client ignored, misused, or wanted for him/herself.

7. Have the client put an X (or nontoxic white-out) on the shoes if he/she now believes that real or imagined bad quality no longer justifies the acting-out behavior.

8. Have the client present each worksheet to the staff or peer whose name is on the bottom line while the client explains how he/she will respect each of the person's gifts in the future. Have the person and staff initial the page when this is done.

9. After all three sheets are completed and presented, have the client briefly discuss, during a group session, experiences associated with the exercise.

10. Have the clients write a gift worksheet about their new and developing good qualities, "gifts," and one nonabusive quality, "the shoes," that others might not like but that doesn't justify others hurting them.

Topic: The temptation song

Purpose: To use music to help clients use the coping skills learned in stage one.

Description: The client will have to cope with deviant urges in settings other than the group. To apply these skills elsewhere, the client needs to remember the skills and learn how they can be applied outside the group. By creating a song about ways to cope with deviant urges in other environments, the client is transferring the skills to other settings.

Directions: 1. Using the worksheet from stage one, the client uses the words "stay away, look away, and get away" to create a song about preventing relapse into deviant sex.

2. The client chooses any familiar tune or rap song.

3. The client writes a copy of the words.

4. The client sings or reads the song to the group.

Topic: Thinking error homework

Purpose: To transfer the client's ability to self-monitor for thinking errors into another environment.

Description: The clients use thinking errors outside the group setting. This task asks the clients to self-monitor their use of thinking errors at other times throughout their day.

Directions: 1. Early in stage two, give each client fourteen blank positive attitude worksheets.

2. The client needs to complete two worksheets per day, for a minimum of seven days. The worksheets are the same as those used in stage one.

3. The client needs to have a staff member read and initial each page on the day it is completed.

4. The client must ask for group time to present the worksheets when all fourteen are completed.

5. The client is asked to explore patterns found and what he learned from this task.

Stage Three: Generalization and Practice

In this stage of treatment, the goal is intermediate transfer. Clients are expected to extend skills and strategies to many situations and environments outside of therapy.

Topic: Positive sexuality role play

Purpose: To transfer client's new knowledge and values about sex into the home environment prior to discharge.

Description: Each client has benefited from spending time in an environment committed to supporting the value of positive sex. For the client to generalize these values from the treatment setting to the home environment, the client must be able to discuss positive sexual values and get support for them from those he will live with in the future. Many families will need education on how to support the positive values the client has learned in treatment.

Directions: 1. During a group therapy session, the client role plays how he thinks family members will respond. The client role plays each family member by using the empty-chair technique. Group members will give suggestions to increase the client's success in this task.
              2. In person or during a teleconference call, the client discusses with family members what he/she has learned about the difference between healthy and deviant sex.
              3. When talking to family members, the client and family are encouraged to discuss any value conflicts.
              4. The client asks family members for support needed to promote future healthy sexual expression by the client.
              5. The client briefly reports to the group the results of this task after it is completed.

Topic: Offense cycle lesson plan
Purpose: To allow client the opportunity to teach his offense cycle to family members to increase accountability and support.
Description: Since most family members ask how they might know if the client is going to offend again, the client needs to share what he has learned about the offense cycle. The materials the client used to learn this concept in stages one and two can be used by the client to teach the family. This puts the responsibility on the client to teach his family how to recognize and respond to the offense cycle.
Directions: 1. The client uses a group session to role play teaching his family the offense cycle. The client asks the group for feedback and suggestions.

2. The client plays a game, role plays, or draws his/her cycle to teach family members in a teleconference call or family session.

3. The client asks his family to give examples of times they recognized he was in this cycle, and discusses how they could intervene.

4. The client requests his family's help and commits to accepting their interventions.

5. The client briefly describes the results of this task with the group members in a therapy session.

Topic: Empathy game

Purpose: To broaden client's support for showing empathy and provide a forum in which the client and his family may discuss this issue.

Description: Some clients come from families that show empathy consistently, while others do not. It is important that all families show empathy for others without devaluing or labeling others. The client and his family members should discuss and agree upon a way for showing empathy.

Directions: 1. The clinician teaches family members the rules of the game.

2. The client and his family play the game for a thirty-minute session.

3. After the session, the client, his family, and the clinician discuss how empathy is shown in the family.

4. The client and his family agree to ways the client and other family members will show empathy in the future.

Topic: Clarification letter

Purpose: To provide an opportunity for the client to provide restitution to one or more of his victims.

Description: Some clients' victims are family members or friends of the family. Whenever the whereabouts of a victim is known, the opportunity to provide clarification to the victim should be offered by the client. The client may need to call the victim's parents or therapist in the presence of his therapist to make this offer. It is always the victim's decision whether or not a clarification session should occur. Whenever there is no opportunity to provide clarification directly, the client can role play the clarification session.

Directions: 1. If the client has an opportunity for a face-to-face clarification meeting with one or more victims, the client must prepare a clarification letter.

2. After completing a clarification letter, the client role plays presenting the letter during a group session, prior to meeting with the victim.

3. The client uses role play to determine how to respect the victim's power. The client prepares for any difficulties group members can anticipate.

4. The client participates in the clarification sessions by reading the letter and answering any of the victim's questions.

5. The client briefly discusses the results of this task in a group session.

Topic: Relapse prevention plan

Purpose: To generalize coping skills by developing a plan that delineates how the skills can be used in the next residential setting.

Description: The coping skills used by the client need to be put in a form that can be understood by everyone who will be providing support and treatment to the client after discharge from the current program. Since the responsibility to avoid relapse falls on the client, the client needs to develop and communicate to others how they can help him use coping skills. This discussion needs to occur with the family, probation officer, and anyone else who can support the client.

Directions: 1. The client completes a relapse prevention plan form.

2. The client reads and discusses it with family members in family session or by teleconference call. (A copy of the plan can be sent to family prior to this phone call.)

Topic: Positive attitudes poster

Purpose: To transfer the use of smart self-talk into the home environment.

Description: To promote the continual use of smart self-talk, the client needs to be taught to seek feedback in any situation where distorted thinking could lead to deviant sex or other abusive behavior. Since many teens use posters to represent what they believe in, the clients create a poster to take home. This is a visual way to transfer smart-talk from the treatment setting to the home setting.

Directions: 1. The client is given art materials to make a poster about the thinking errors and smart self-talk. The client works on the poster during free time, not during group.

2. The client presents the poster in a family session and teaches family members about the thinking errors and smart self-talk, and why these issues are important.

3. The client and family discuss how they can

hold the client accountable for thinking errors and support the client's attempts to use smart self-talk.

4. The client gives the poster to the family to put on the client's wall to prepare for homecoming.

5. The client briefly shares the results of this task with the group.

Stage Four: Transition Planning

When a client leaves a residential center, he or she usually experiences a regression. Since clients in this program are sex offenders, a regression may entail a re-offense. This stage of treatment is designed to prevent that occurrence.

Topic: Schedule

Purpose: To make client's transition smoother by pre-planning how time will be spent to avoid high-risk situations and other threats to self-control.

Description: Many clients state that they tend to fantasize and plan deviant sex in response to boredom or unstructured time. At other times, due to poor planning, they may find themselves in a situation that promotes sexual acting out. Regardless of how it comes to pass, high-risk situations threaten relapse, and consequently the situations should be avoided. That is why clients develop schedules. The schedule needs to be realistic. It needs to be revised with a trusted adult so clients can update it as necessary. Most of all, the schedule needs to be used to keep the clients out of high-risk situations.

Directions: 1. The client completes a schedule of time to be spent at the home or at the discharge placement. This includes time the client spends at school, work, sports, and other activities.

2. The client fills out a schedule in ink or marker according to current realistic plans. The client can use a pencil to write in how he/she hopes activities will change; for example, if the client hopes to get a job or be selected for a sports team, this can be penciled in until it is a reality.

3. A copy of this schedule is sent to the family and the client's outpatient therapist to approve the schedule and assess the reality of the client's plans before the client is discharged.

Topic: Transition plans

Purpose: To facilitate a smooth transition from treatment.

Description: To move on to a new phase of life, a person must separate from a current phase. The separation process involves the grief over change. This grieving process often includes a time of reminiscing about the current phase. This can sometimes lead to a regression to old behaviors. This regression may serve the purpose of avoiding the task of separation. If this process is anticipated, the regression may be diminished. Many clients state that they had little intimacy with same-age peers prior to treatment. For many clients this is the first time they will face separation from such close relationships. Separation also requires the person to consider the possibility of new relationships in the future. This might be a fear-inducing experience for some clients.

Directions: 1. The client completes the transition plan in writing outside group or opts to be interviewed by the group, according to questions on this sheet in one of the client's last sessions.

2. The client's answers are discussed and an attempt is made to help the client achieve a full separation from staff and peers.

5

Program Development: The Renaissance Program

Although the residential treatment center is the ideal setting for treating the neurologically impaired juvenile sex offender, not all sex offenders placed in a residential center will have neurological impairments. Just as it would be inappropriate to require the neurologically impaired juvenile sex offender to complete a treatment program not modified to compensate for the deficit resulting from the neurological impairment, it would be inappropriate to require the neurologically intact juvenile sex offender to adhere to a program that is tailored to meet the needs of the neurologically impaired client. Consequently, a treatment program designed for use with non-neurologically impaired clients is needed.

There is a variety of programs and manuals that could be used to establish a sex offender treatment program at a residential facility. There are typically great differences between programs in terms of techniques, terminology, and long-term treatment goals. It is difficult to maintain two sex offender treatment programs at a facility if they are too dissimilar. On the other hand, by having two programs that are based on similar concepts and requirements, it would be easier to maintain program requirements across the campus. Furthermore, similarity between the programs would permit clinicians to cross over from one program to another with a minimum of change, thereby minimizing the staff shortages that are so common in the field of contemporary residential treatment.

The program for the neurologically intact juvenile sex offender designed to coexist at a facility where the Bridges Program is used is known as the Renaissance Program. The underlying theme of this program is that clients will experience a rebirth. Specifically, it is expected that clients will enter the program in a state of mind that promotes deviant sexual behavior. It is expected that through a series of therapeutic tasks clients will shun their deviant mind set and experience a cognitive awakening that results in positive, prosocial behavior.

The client workbook for the Renaissance Program contains descriptions of all the therapeutic tasks that a client must complete in order to graduate from the program (see Appendix B). For each therapeutic task listed in the client workbook, a rationale is provided to explain why the task is included as a part of the treatment program. Each task is described in detail. It is likely that clients and clinicians alike will find the workbook "user friendly." Still, the workbook is lacking in one respect: while it provides a wealth of detailed information, it is not designed to provide an overview of the course of treatment. This chapter provides such an overview. It begins with an explanation of why the cognitive-behavioral approach was selected as the primary methodology of the treatment program. Then the sequence of treatment interventions is discussed. Experience has suggested that a particular sequence of therapeutic tasks is most often associated with successful program outcome. The components of the treatment program are also discussed. Finally, the therapeutic modalities, such as group and family therapy, and methods for coordinating these treatment modalities are discussed.

COGNITIVE-BEHAVIORAL APPROACH

The cognitive-behavioral approach is based upon the assumption that cognitions determine emotions and behavior.

Further, it is assumed that relatively fixed patterns of thinking result in fixed emotional and behavior patterns. Cognitive-behavioral therapy is primarily an issue of changing the client's thought patterns. It is argued that changes in the person's thinking will result in altered emotions and behaviors.

There are many methods associated with the cognitive-behavioral approach. All methods share one common goal: eliminate undesirable cognitions and teach adaptive cognitions. Some of the methods commonly used in the cognitive behavioral approach include teaching, assertiveness training, behavioral contracting, role playing, relapse prevention, and guided group interaction. As with other approaches, cognitive behavioral techniques can be used in individual or group therapy.

A recent nationwide survey of juvenile sex offender treatment programs revealed that the cognitive-behavioral approach is currently the most widely utilized approach when dealing with juvenile sex offenders (Knopp et al. 1992). Table 5-1 gives the results of the nationwide survey.

As can be seen by this survey, the cognitive-behavioral approach is the most commonly used treatment model, with 43 percent. However, if a more liberal definition of cognitive-behavioral treatment is used, then any treatment program

Table 5-1.
Nationwide Survey of Treatment Models Used by Juvenile Sex Offenders Treatment Programs

Treatment Model	N	%
Cognitive-behavioral	314	43
Psychosocial-educational	196	27
Relapse prevention	95	13
Psychotherapeutic	74	10
Family systems	21	3
Sexual-addictive	8	1
Behavioral	6	1
Psychoanalytic	2	0
Biomedical	0	0
Other	19	3

that relies on teaching new skills or attitudes could be included in the cognitive-behavioral category. Of the programs listed in Table 5-1, three additional programs are eligible to be included in the cognitive-behavioral category: psychosocial-educational, relapse prevention, and behavioral. When these treatment models are included in the cognitive-behavioral category, the percentage of programs employing the cognitive-behavioral model is approximately 84 percent. Obviously, the cognitive-behavioral approach is unparalleled in the treatment of juvenile sex offenders.

The cognitive-behavioral approach is widely used because it has proved to reduce recidivism among all types of juvenile and adult offenders, including sex offenders. Even a cursory review of the rehabilitation literature supports the contention that cognitive-behavioral treatment reduces recidivism. Consider the following summary of the research findings regarding interventions that have demonstrated the ability to reduce recidivism (Garrett 1985; Gendreau and Ross 1979, 1984, 1987):

1. Family therapy with parents and delinquents that teaches parents communication and discipline skills.
2. Token economies that offer reward for prosocial behavior.
3. Behavioral contracting designed to reward prosocial behavior.
4. Role playing designed to teach prosocial skills (e.g., assertiveness).
5. Guided group interaction in which a prosocial facilitator encourages peers to confront and eliminate delinquent thinking.
6. Self-examination techniques designed to detect and eliminate criminogenic thoughts.
7. Education programs that teach problem solving and moral reasoning.

These interventions have proven to reduce re-offense rates among all types of delinquent and adult offenders. These same techniques are associated with positive outcomes in the treatment of juvenile sex offenders (Knopp 1982). Each of the seven interventions is designed to alter the client's thinking pattern. But what about the techniques that do not attempt to alter the client's cognitive style? Are these techniques effective?

The correctional rehabilitation research is replete with studies of failed programs. The literature is amply clear regarding the types of treatment programs that result in failure to reduce recidivism. Here is a summary of treatment approaches most likely to fail to reduce recidivism:

1. Counseling based on the notion that the delinquent wants to change or self-actualize.
2. Self-help groups in which delinquents control the topics of discussion and the manner in which issues are discussed.
3. Any counseling that is nondirective (e.g., Rogerian or psychoanalytic).
4. Programs based upon a medical model (i.e., the delinquent acts as he does due to a disease process).
5. Behavior programs that give rewards for the absence of behavior, not for increased use of prosocial behavior.
6. Failure to confront and neutralize delinquent behavior in sessions and throughout the program.
7. Programs that do not directly address the misconduct that resulted in the client's placement in the program.

Just as the treatment interventions that are effective share a common theme, the treatment programs that are ineffective all seem to fail to confront the criminogenic thoughts and behaviors. Without confronting, and to some degree limiting criminogenic thoughts, the offender has no reason to change. It is only when the clinician actively confronts the offender and eliminates the offender's ability to meet his needs through delinquent behavior that the offender begins to use prosocial behavior.

Even though the research is quite clear, it would appear that some treatment programs use techniques that in effect promote treatment failure. Keeping in mind the list of interventions that are associated with failure, consider the treatment models listed in Table 5–1. There are two treatment models that are certainly inappropriate to use with juvenile sex offenders: the sexual-addictive and the psychoanalytic models. A little over 1 percent of the programs included in the nationwide survey report using one of these treatment models. It is somewhat of a relief that so few programs rely on these models. Yet, use of these models is associated with program failure. Unfortunately, failure to effectively treat the juvenile sex offender results in further sexual misconduct and an increase in victims. Thus, any use of these treatment models is costly and should not be tolerated.

Despite the well-documented ineffectiveness of the psychoanalytic and addictive models, it is unlikely that these models will be readily dispatched. The psychoanalytic model is the oldest and most revered of treatment models. It is effective in some treatment areas, but not in correctional rehabilitation. Its status as the original treatment model may provide enough of a defense for those who would use the psychoanalytic approach with juvenile sex offenders.

The addiction model of sex offending may be the most resilient model in the field because it derives its strength from two areas. First, sex offenders prefer to be treated under the addiction model because it is based upon the notion that they are "powerless" over their sexual behavior. There may be nothing more countertherapeutic than to allow a sex offender to avoid personal responsibility for sexual misconduct. The addiction model affords the offender this opportunity. Second, the addiction model is based on self-help. Again, this seems quite desirable to the sex offender but that is not the real source of its resiliency. Self-help groups are not facilitated by paid professionals. Consequently, self-help groups are vastly less expensive than other forms of treatment. This is the real source of resiliency of the addiction model: it costs less. In these times of shrinking treatment budgets, the addiction model is very appealing to many. Unfortunately, the result of the addiction model is an increase in victims because it does not reduce re-offenses rates.

Overall, it is not difficult to select an effective treatment model to use with the juvenile sex offender. Certain pitfalls must be avoided, for example, seeking the least expensive approach. By adhering to the findings in the more than thirty years of correctional rehabilitation research, it is possible to develop a treatment program based on interventions and techniques that are associated with reduced re-offense rates. In development of the Renaissance Program, the correctional rehabilitation research did serve as the foundation, and consequently a cognitive-behavioral approach was selected as the basis for the program.

SEQUENCE OF TREATMENT

Use of the cognitive behavioral approach ensures the potential for program success. Still, there is the matter of selecting specific treatment interventions and arranging these interventions in a temporal sequence that maximizes their effectiveness.

Selection of interventions to be used in a juvenile sex offender program should be based upon the outcomes literature, that is, on their ability to reduce recidivism. As discussed in the preceding section, interventions that teach prosocial skills or teach control of deviant thoughts and behaviors are effective in reducing re-offense. There is an advantage in selecting interventions known to be effective: treatment is expedited.

Another way to expedite treatment is to select interventions based upon a conceptualization about how clients change during treatment. In the Renaissance Program, it is assumed clients change as a result of a three-step process:

Self-Awareness → Self-Monitoring → Self-Control

Self-awareness is achieved when the client reduces denial and admits to the criminogenic thoughts and planning that precede deviant sexual behavior. Self-monitoring is a matter of being able to recognize behavioral precursors to sexual misconduct, for example, "grooming." Self-control refers to the cognitive and behavioral strategies that eliminate the precursor to sexual misconduct and the actual sexual misconduct itself.

Table 5-2 depicts the strategy used to identify the treatment interventions that comprise the Renaissance Program. Notice that interventions aim to alter the client's thinking and behavior, in keeping with the cognitive behavioral approach. Also notice that each of the interventions serves to address one of the three components of the change process.

Interventions are designed to alter both the client's thinking and behavior. For the most part, self-awareness and

Table 5-2.
Matrix for Selecting Therapeutic Interventions

	Thinking	*Behavior*
Self-awareness	Thinking errors Denial Empathy for others	Offense cycle Grooming
Self-monitoring	Seemingly unimportant decisions	High-risk situations
Self-control	Assertiveness Positive sexual image Punishment-scene covert sensitizations Planning	Avoidance techniques Escape techniques

self-monitoring focus upon deviant thoughts and behaviors. The aim is to teach clients how to recognize and eliminate deviant thoughts before the thoughts are manifested in behavior. Being aware of one's deviant strivings is only part of the solution. The client is expected to respond to his deviant strivings by using self-control. In Table 5–2, the row pertaining to self-control reveals the techniques used to teach clients how to respond to deviant thoughts and behaviors. Much of self-control is a matter of avoiding or escaping situations that promote deviant sexual behavior. Clients are also expected to learn to channel their sexuality into acceptable forms of sexual behavior, for example, prosocial skills, assertiveness, and positive sexuality.

Overall, the interventions that comprise the Renaissance Program were selected on the basis of their ability to enhance the client's self-awareness, self-monitoring, and self-control. While it is known that these interventions can have impact on the client, there is still the matter of arranging these interventions in the most efficacious sequence.

Therapy is a process that unfolds over time. Different issues are salient at different points in the treatment process. To achieve maximum impact, treatment interventions should be arranged in a manner that makes maximum use of the limited time available for treatment. Like other human endeavors, the therapy process may be viewed as an activity with a beginning, middle, and end. The relevant issues in therapy change as the client moves from one phase of treatment to the next.

During the beginning phase of sex offender treatment, the client is typically concerned with perpetuating his secretiveness. The client can be expected to be reluctant to discuss his deviant sexual behavior. It is even more unlikely that the client will admit to deviant thoughts or fantasies. Many times the client's reluctance to discuss his sexual misconduct is construed as denial. In many respects, denial may be an accurate depiction of the client's behavior. Yet, it is important to remember that the client is a sex offender. The client used secretiveness as a method to gain access to control his victim. For the sex offender, secretiveness is synonymous with control. When the client enters treatment, he feels out of control. Hence, the client clings to his secretiveness as if he were clinging to the last shreds of control in his life.

Two things need to happen at the beginning of treatment to assist the client. First, the client should undergo an orientation training designed to teach him how to be a success in treatment. The juvenile sex offender wants to be in control. He may use secretiveness to be in control, until he learns a different method of maintaining control. It should not be assumed that the client knows how to behave in a treatment program. Instead, he should be taught how to behave. Furthermore, he should be encouraged to feel in control by use of positive therapy skills, not secretiveness.

While being urged to use positive therapy skills, the client should be made to feel uncomfortable about being secretive. All clients in the beginning phase of treatment should be given the expectation that they will talk about their sexual misconduct in an open, honest manner. Toward this end, the client is given the assignment of writing a description of the sexual misconduct that resulted in his being placed in a sex offender treatment program, and sharing his written account with staff, his peers, and his family. In doing so, the client relinquishes secretiveness about his sexual deviance but he is allowed to achieve self-control, perhaps even self-esteem, by using the therapy skills that were taught in orientation.

As the client openly admits to his sexual deviance, he moves from the beginning phase of treatment to the middle phase, the longest and most complicated phase. In juvenile sex offender treatment, two issues consume the efforts of the client and the clinician: behavioral patterns and emotional residue. The treatment efforts are designed to help the client develop self-awareness about his own personal pattern of sexual acting out. The client learns that he does indeed follow a specific pattern of sexual misconduct and that both behavioral and cognitive events precede and follow the deviant sexual act. A premium is placed on being able to recognize the precursors of sexual misconduct and take steps to avoid engaging in deviant sexual behavior.

With regard to emotional residue, the client must attend to the emotional fallout that he created when he harmed his victim(s). This is also the time at which the client addresses the emotional reactions that he experiences in response to abuse he has suffered. Most juvenile sex offenders will have experienced some form of abuse or neglect during their lives, usually more physical abuse than sexual abuse. Nonetheless, abuse does cause the emotional residue that the client must address.

The issue of sequencing is no more important than when the topic of the client's own abuse is addressed. Some treatment providers have tried to address the client's own abuse prior to addressing the abuse that the client perpetrated. If one considers the etiology of the client's sexual deviance to be his own abuse, then addressing the client's experience as a victim before addressing his behavior as a perpetrator makes sense. However, actual experience with juvenile sex offenders has proven this approach to be unwise. When the clinician addresses the client's experience as a victim first, the client will hide behind the victim persona in an effort to avoid being held accountable for the sexual misconduct that he perpetrated. As a result of this defensiveness, treatment is prolonged.

Ironically, if treatment is sequenced such that the client's experiences as victim are dealt with after his perpetration behavior has been addressed, treatment is expedited. It seems as if the client becomes somewhat of an expert on the characteristics of a perpetrator by dealing with his own perpetration issues. The client comes to accept that the perpetrator is responsible for the sexual misconduct and the victim is not to blame. This awareness that the victim is not to blame seems to be particularly helpful to the client when the client is considering his experiences as victim of abuse. Just as he is taught to hold himself strictly accountable for his behavior as a perpetrator, he is encouraged to recognize that the person who perpetrated abuse against him is responsible for that abuse. It seems as if the knowledge gained from dealing with his issues as a perpetrator assists the client in working through the experience of being a victim.

The end phase of treatment begins when the client appears to have gained control over deviant urges and increased his ability to modulate and express emotions. The primary issue of the end phase of treatment is maintaining the positive changes that resulted from the work done in the previous two phases. In contemporary treatment of juvenile sex offenders, this issue is often referred to as relapse prevention.

There are many interventions that can be used to help clients maintain positive changes. Two of the more common techniques are role play and planning. Role play serves to reduce relapse by allowing the client to practice prosocial skills that could prevent relapse. If relapse is conceptualized as the result of deviant urges that overwhelm the person's skills, then relapse prevention becomes a matter of strengthening the client's skills such that few, if any, deviant urges could overwhelm the skills. Role play seems to strengthen prosocial skills.

Planning facilitates relapse prevention in two ways. First, planning forces the client to transfer skills learned in therapy to situations outside therapy. The result is that prosocial skills generalize, and consequently these skills become available to the client in a variety of situations. Second, planning allows the client to develop a response to stressors before the stress arrives. It is not a matter of whether or not a person will experience stress. It is a matter of how much stress will occur and what a person does in response to the stress. Consequently, it is important to plan for stress and hone these plans during periods of calm. The proactive person always copes more effectively than the reactive person.

Overall, therapeutic interventions are most effective when used in proper sequence. Table 5-3 summarizes the recommended sequence. The Renaissance Program follows a specific sequence of therapeutic interventions. This sequence is delineated in the stages of treatment, the temporal order of therapeutic interventions that corresponds to the various phases and issues that a client experiences. The goal of sequencing treatment interventions is to expedite treatment while ensuring treatment effectiveness.

TREATMENT MODALITIES

As with most programs in residential treatment centers, a juvenile sex offender treatment program should take advantage of varied treatment modalities. The juvenile sex-offending client should become involved in group therapy,

Table 5-3.
Issues and Interventions for Each Phase of Treatment

Phase	Issue	Intervention
Beginning	Denial Secretiveness Control	Orientation Deviant sex worksheet
Middle	Behavioral patterns Cognitive precursors Self-control Emotional residue	Offense cycle worksheet Positive and deviant sex Covert sensitization Victim story Clarification letter
End	Skill maintenance Gaining perspective Termination	ACE worksheet Relapse prevention Healthy sexual expression Transition plan

individual therapy, family therapy, psychoeducational classes, and adjunctive therapies. While the juvenile sex-offending client can benefit from participating in all of these modalities, the more each modality is tailored to meet the needs of the client the more the client will benefit. There are guidelines for using each of these modalities with juvenile sex offenders.

Group Therapy

The clinician cannot use a nondirective approach when dealing with juvenile sex offenders. This is particularly true with regard to group therapy. The juvenile sex offender in a group session with a nondirective clinician will receive little therapy. The delinquent will perceive the nondirective clinician as weak. The sex offender views the world in terms of winners and losers, and he will associate the therapist's passivity with being a loser. The client will find little motivation to relinquish his exploitive ways, and, above all, he will refuse to adopt a prosocial stance if being prosocial means being weak, like the clinician.

The solution is not for the clinician to be harsh and controlling. Rather, the solution is to provide structure and direction. Much structure is inherent in the client workbook. Clients know that they must complete the therapeutic tasks in this workbook if they are to graduate from the program. Still, the workbook is not enough to structure the time spent in the group therapy session. Therefore, it is necessary that the clinician structure these sessions.

Ferrara (1992) recommends that each group therapy session follow a three-step process: layout, problem solving, and conclusion. Each step is designed to provide a framework within which the client can accomplish necessary therapeutic goals.

The layout, used at the beginning of a group session, is a

self-report — clients report on their behavior since the last group therapy session. The layout typically requires the client to state his name and admit to deviant sexual behavior. Oftentimes the client is required to list all victims and all deviant behaviors in his layout. Clients are also expected to reveal any violations of the treatment contract they have committed since the last session. The layout concludes with the client identifying the issue that he would like to address in treatment. The following is a typical layout:

> "My name is Tony. I am a sex offender. I raped my sister by placing my finger in her vagina. I have also exposed myself. Since the last group I violated the rule about not looking down female blouses twice. My topic for today is the offense cycle worksheet."

Many goals are accomplished merely by starting a group session with a layout. First, the client's desire to remain secretive about his sexual misconduct is undermined. The client must admit he has engaged in sexual misconduct. Not only that, he must describe the sexual acting out that resulted in his being placed in a sex offender treatment program, and he must identify any other victims. Second, the client must self-report rule violations. Most juvenile sex offenders are not self-critical, but the layout requires that the client start each group session by being self-critical. Finally, the client is required to select a topic to discuss. The topic that the client selects should pertain to his own treatment, for example, a therapeutic task from the client workbook. The requirement of having a personal agenda item to discuss each group session implies that the client attends group therapy to receive help.

After layouts are completed, a client is permitted to present his topic. The client who presents a topic is encouraged to receive help, that is, to be open to feedback from peers. The clients who listen as a peer self-discloses are encouraged to give help, that is, to listen and be prepared to offer feedback. In a well-functioning group, the clinician should have to speak very little. Instead, the group members should offer most of the feedback. When the members of a group do not actively give or receive help, the clinician can best spend his/her time by teaching the clients how to give and receive help.

The group session should conclude with the clinician summarizing the events that transpired during the session. This is an ideal time to teach the clients how to give and receive help. When possible, the clinician should individually praise group members who fulfilled the members' role, that is, to give or receive help. Social praise is a powerful reinforcer.

This three-step group process is not the only method for providing directive group therapy. There are many ways to structure the group therapy session. The important issue is that the session must be structured or the clients will structure it themselves, that is, they will act delinquent and they will derive little benefit from being in the session.

Individual Therapy

In most juvenile sex offender treatment programs, group therapy is viewed as the primary treatment modality, and has been found to be far more effective than individual therapy when dealing with juvenile delinquents (Agee and McWilliams 1984). This does not mean that individual therapy should not be used. Rather, it suggests that individual therapy should be used carefully.

To the extent possible, individual therapy should be used to support group therapy. One easy method for accomplishing this goal is to use individual therapy to work on assignments from the client workbook. Assignments that are completed in individual therapy can be presented in a group therapy session. Clients may feel more confident when presenting assignments if they first had the opportunity to work on the assignment in individual therapy.

It should be noted that individual therapy is one setting in which splitting may occur. The client in individual therapy is very likely to try to split the individual therapist from the other members of the treatment team (e.g., "I trust you so I'll tell you something but I do not want the other staff to know"). Most attempts at splitting can be readily defeated by reminding the client of the treatment contract, that is, what a client tells one staff member, he tells all staff members.

Family Therapy

If the client is to return home upon completing treatment, then family therapy is a necessity. Family therapy can be used to prepare the family to accept the client after the client has changed as a result of therapy. In the family systems approach, it is well known that changes in one part of the family system affects all other parts of the family system. Some family therapists have noted that families unprepared for the changes in a client will try to undo the changes that the client has made, even if the changes are for the better. Consequently the main goal of family therapy should be to prepare the family to accept the client back into the family system after the client has changed.

The most straightforward method of preparing the family for the changes resulting from treatment is to permit the client to present to the family completed assignments from the client workbook. In fact, it may be best for the client to present assignments as he completes them rather than presenting all worksheets toward the end of treatment. By slowly and methodically introducing assignments into family therapy, clinicians can help the family deal with issues in the same sequence and time frame as the client. This gives the family time to address and process issues in depth. Most importantly, it affords the family more time to change.

Psychoeducational Training

Even though juvenile sex offenders are skillful in exploiting others, it should not be assumed that they are equally skillful in being prosocial. To the contrary, it appears that the more skilled the youth is in being exploitive, the less likely he/she is to have prosocial skills (Goldstein 1988). Therefore, if clients are expected to be prosocial, they must be taught the prosocial skills they are expected to use.

There are several specific areas in which juvenile sex offenders could benefit from skills training. Any treatment program hoping to increase the juvenile sex offender's prosocial behavior should, at a minimum, address the following issues: thinking errors, aggression control, self-esteem, human sexuality, relationship issues, and problem solving. The manner in which these topics are addressed is also important.

When learning social skills, clients should be exposed to didactic information and they should be allowed to practice new skills. Didactic information should be presented in a lecture format. The clinician should instruct the clients in such a way that a social skill is defined and examples are provided. Then, the clients should be allowed to practice the skill during training. This can be most easily achieved by conducting role plays during psychoeducational sessions. However, training should not be restricted to the training sessions. Clients should be given homework assignments that require them to practice the skills in other settings, for example, the dorm or classroom. At least some segment of the training sessions should be dedicated to debriefing homework assignments. The clinician should look for opportunities to bolster the client's sense of accomplishment when he experiences some success in using social skills.

Adjunctive Therapies

The adjunctive therapies include art therapy, music therapy, theater arts, and other expressive therapies. By themselves, these therapies are inadequate for treating juvenile sex offenders. However, when used in conjunction with cognitive-behavioral interventions, their impact can be beneficial.

Cognitive-behavioral interventions are decidedly cerebral—the client is required to analyze and use deductive reasoning. With enough experience using these techniques, a client may develop defenses that effectively defeat his attempts to analyze and become more self-aware. By switching to an alternative method of developing self-awareness, the client may circumvent his own defenses and uncover previously blocked material.

Whereas cognitive-behavioral interventions promote self-awareness through analysis, adjunctive therapies promote self-awareness through intuition and sensing. It might be useful to think of the dichotomy of functions in the right and left hemispheres of the brain. The left hemisphere is the locus of language and logic. The right hemisphere supports functions that are more intuitive and synthetic. Cognitive-behavioral techniques require clients to use their left hemisphere, and adjunctive therapies challenge clients to use their right hemisphere. Presumably, defenses designed to defeat left hemispheric functions are ineffective with right hemispheric functions, thus allowing clients to gain access to previously defended material.

CONCLUSIONS

It seems like there is never enough time to treat a client. Therefore, it is essential that there be no wasted effort in treatment. When treating the juvenile sex offender, the efficient program will be based upon the cognitive-behavioral treatment approach. Furthermore, great care will be taken to usher the client through a predetermined sequence of treatment events. To further enhance the effectiveness of treatment, the client should be required to participate in a variety of treatment modalities. However, the primacy of group therapy should be recognized and all other treatment modalities should be orchestrated to support group therapy.

6

Creating a Therapeutic Milieu

The victims of juvenile sex offenders are usually younger and to some degree defenseless. But the juvenile sex offender is not limited to exploiting younger, more vulnerable victims. The juvenile sex offender has at his disposal a repertoire of skills and ploys that permit him to exploit others in sexual and nonsexual ways.

Just because the juvenile sex offender is placed in a residential facility, the exploitive behavior does not cease. He looks for opportunities to exploit others in a therapeutic residential environment just as he looked for opportunities to exploit others prior to being placed in a secure setting. Who is it that these young clients may try to exploit? The answer is not surprising: anybody in his current environment.

Given the fact that juvenile sex offenders do continue their exploitive behaviors even after placed in a therapeutic environment, the effective treatment program will include the means to manage this behavior. This chapter discusses creating a safe environment in which offenders' opportunities to use exploitive behavior are minimized. The issues discussed are countertransference, splitting, deception, delinquent games, and finally the treatment contract, the primary tool used to bring exploitive behavior into the therapeutic arena.

COUNTERTRANSFERENCE

Countertransference refers to the clinician's thoughts and feelings about the client that interfere with the orderly delivery of treatment services. Not all thoughts and feelings experienced by clinicians are countertransference. Only those reactions that impede the clinician's ability to act responsibly are considered countertransference.

It might be useful to consider a continuum of responses that a clinician, or direct care staff, might have in response to the juvenile sex offender client. At one end of the continuum, there is the permissive accepting response. At the other end is the strict, punishing response. The centerpoint of the continuum is a position of balance and flexibility. It is proposed that the centerpoint is the therapeutic position and the polar positions are countertransference.

The permissive approach to juvenile sex offenders has been tried and it has failed (Izzo and Ross 1990). In the permissive approach, the clinician uses the rationale: "These clients would not have done what they did if only someone had loved them. So I will love and accept them." Examination of the effects of this approach has revealed that juvenile delinquents who are treated with unconditional positive regard do not relinquish their delinquent ways (Garrett 1985).

Assuming that a clinician is aware that uncritical acceptance is not appropriate, the question arises: Why would a clinician use this approach? Frequently, the answer lies in the clinician's ability to accept his/her own aggressive impulses. The clinician who recognizes the exploitive, aggressive behavior in others must also be capable of recognizing these same impulses in him/herself. Some clinicians have dealt with these impulses by repression or denial. In the absence of these aggressive impulses, the clinician may feel a pervasive sense of well-being. To preserve their own sense of well-being, these clinicians must assume that other people, even their clients, are just like them, that is, full of good and devoid of aggression. Treatment then becomes a matter of scraping away the crusty nastiness so the wholesome individual underneath can be exposed. The clinician with this form of countertransference tends to be permissive and accepting of the client and confrontation is avoided.

This type of countertransference is easy to recognize. This clinician will often engage in one or more of the following behaviors:

1. Find reasons to avoid giving consequences to clients who act out.
2. Recommend that punishment and negative reinforcement not be used.
3. Develop theories of juvenile sex-offending behavior that explain it as harmless misguided behavior or once-in-a-lifetime experimental behavior.
4. Make indirect comments designed to make colleagues feel guilty for enforcing rules.

Perhaps one of the most unique aspects of working with neurologically impaired juvenile sex offenders is that a novel rationale can be used to support the permissive approach — for example, "These youths have frontal lobe damage so it will be of no avail to confront them since they cannot learn from negative feedback." This rationale is little more than a clinical hypothesis that is easily dismissed when put to a critical test. Neurologically impaired youths do respond to negative feedback and all one has to do to know this is use negative feedback and observe the effect.

At the other end of the continuum of countertransference is the strict, punishing approach. In this approach, the clinician uses this rationale: "These clients are dangerous so I should use every tool at my disposal to neutralize them." As with the permissive approach, the strict approach has also been found to be ineffective in helping juvenile delinquents become more prosocial (Izzo and Ross 1990). This finding should come as no surprise. After all, the strict approach will inevitably result in a power struggle between the clinician and the client. The strength of the juvenile sex offender lies in his ability to engage in power struggles. In fact, there is nothing that a juvenile sex offender will not do to win a power struggle. On the other hand, the clinician is constrained by legal and ethical standards, and consequently the clinician is unable to escalate or engage in power struggles in the same unbridled manner as the client. Hence, the strict approach does not promote change on behalf of clients, it solidifies their delinquent skills.

The underlying countertransference issues in the strict approach is more complex than the countertransference associated with the permissive approach. The strict countertransference typically arises from one of two sources: fear of aggression or narcissism. The clinician who experiences the fear-of-aggression countertransference actually fears the clients. This clinician will use the strict approach as a preemptive strike: get the client before the client gets me. With regard to narcissism, the clinician is engaged in competition with the client. The clinician knows that the client will be aggressive and exploitive. The clinician challenges himself to recognize and defeat every manipulative ploy, even before it happens. This clinician seems to be operating on the notion that success means never having been manipulated by the client.

The strict countertransference is easy to recognize. The clinician who has succumbed to this form of countertransference may exhibit one or more of the following behaviors:

1. Fails to show compassion or caring for the clients.
2. Develops punitive programs that do not afford clients the opportunity to develop positive self-worth.
3. Is unwilling to lift restrictions for a client even when the client attains goal behaviors.

4. Uses the formal system of consequences to "break the spirit" of the client.
5. Uses the formal system of consequences for revenge against clients who have successfully exploited or manipulated staff or other clients.
6. Reports that he/she has never been conned or manipulated or can recognize all such behavior before it happens.
7. Places him/herself in dangerous situations with clients and refuses to recognize the danger.

The clinician with strict countertransference is easy for the client to manipulate. Most clients would recognize this person as vulnerable. It is likely that the excessively strict clinician is in many ways reminiscent of the previous authority figures in the client's life. The client has developed skills to defeat this type of authority figure. The clinician who is strict and punitive is walking straight into the strength of the client's defenses.

There is a balance that can be struck when dealing with the juvenile sex-offending client. This approach entails some permissiveness and some strictness, each in moderation. The key to working with the juvenile sex-offending client is for the clinician to be flexible enough to match interventions to the client's behavior. When the client is troubled and confused, the clinician needs to be empathic and supportive. When the client is aggressive and exploitive, the clinician must respond with confrontation and, if necessary, sanctions. The therapeutic approach requires a dynamic flexibility on the part of the clinician in which the clinician does not restrict him/herself to one manner of intervening. Nor does the clinician go too far in being either permissive or strict.

Ferrara (1992) has suggested that there are identifiable characteristics of clinicians who are effective with these types of client. Five characteristics were identified:

Committed — The clinician is intrinsically motivated and does not need the acceptance or friendship of clients.

Responsible — The clinician is a role model of prosocial behavior and behavior in moderation.

Intense — The clinician pursues his/her work with an intensity that reflects self-motivation and a desire to succeed.

Skeptical — A nonjudgmental stance is used in which the clinician neither accepts nor rejects the client's verbalization; that is, the clinician is always curious and probing.

Leadership — The clinician advocates and rewards prosocial behavior and confronts and gives consequences to exploitive or aggressive behavior.

In the noncountertransferential approach, the clinician is both accepting and confrontive. The clinician does not expect to find a self-actualized, prosocial being under the crusty exterior of pain and abuse. Rather, the clinician should realize that the client can be aggressive and exploitive, and only by the clinician's confronting these negative characteristics and teaching prosocial behaviors will the client improve. Conversely, the clinician must not view the client as unmitigated and pure trouble that needs to be boxed up and controlled. There is only one aspect of the client's behavior that needs to be confronted: the harmful behavior. The clinician must be able to teach and support in response to deficits, and confront in response to harmful behavior. The effective clinician is flexible and responsive. The clinician with countertransferential issues is rigid and ineffective. O'Connel and colleagues (1990) offer guidelines for selecting therapists for sex offenders.

GUIDING PRINCIPLES

Finding a therapeutic approach is difficult enough on an individual basis but developing and maintaining a consistent therapeutic approach on a treatment team is even more difficult. It seems as if the difficulties associated with countertransference are compounded exponentially with the addition of each member to the treatment team. The client is not ignorant of the problems associated with maintaining a consistent team approach. In fact, many clients try to exploit this intrinsic weakness, and this behavior is known as splitting.

Splitting occurs when a client promotes and exploits differences that occur naturally among treatment team members. Splitting is especially effective when staff have not recognized and do not control their own countertransference. When treatment team members do not recognize their own countertransference, then each time they deal with a client they are dealing with two types of behavior: the client's behavior and their countertransference. Since no single solution can contend with the twofold problem, it is difficult for treatment team members to resolve splits.

To effectively deal with splitting, a preventative approach should be utilized. Many of the problems associated with splitting could be avoided by ensuring that treatment team members have a well-articulated set of guiding principles. Conversely, it is known that treatment programs in which staff do not use or support a common philosophy fail to reduce the re-offense rate of the offenders who receive treatment (Gendreau and Ross 1984).

The treatment team should develop a set of guiding principles. These principles should be established in the treatment team setting. All staff should be permitted to provide input into the development of these principles. Once the principles have been established, all treatment team members should adhere to the principles when resolving issues about clients. As new treatment team members join the staff, they should be inculcated in these principles. From time to time, the principles should be evaluated and revised as necessary.

There are four guiding principles that a treatment team should address. The parameters associated with each of these guiding principles is discussed below. Each treatment team would need to add the specific details from its setting to each of the principles.

Philosophy

A treatment team philosophy should articulate assumptions about the clients and the treatment necessary to rehabilitate these clients. When working with juvenile sex offenders it is necessary to describe these clients in terms of their delinquent and developmental characteristics. Discussion of the treatment approach should address the heart of the permissive versus strict issue in staff responses.

Goals

Surprisingly, there is often little agreement about the objectives of treatment. Perhaps this is the result of the different disciplines and different backgrounds of the persons composing the treatment team. Still, it is important that everyone on the treatment team work toward a common goal. Each treatment team should develop multiple goals for its program. It is typical for a program to have between three and ten goals. Goals should refer to client behavior in the program and after completing the program. Goals referring to in-program client behavior should address how the client behaves in therapy, in the dorm, and in school.

Staff Role

The behavior expected of staff should be specified. The preceding section on countertransference could provide the basis of discussion. Ideally, the staff role should describe how staff should behave. It may be useful to identify three to seven behaviors staff are expected (or required) to exhibit.

Client's Role

Often overlooked are the expectations that staff has for clients. It is important to clearly articulate expectations to clients in positive terms, that is, behaviors that the client can exhibit. Most programs dealing with juvenile sex offenders usually expect clients to give help and receive help. The behavioral expectations of clients should form the basis of the program's level system and discipline system.

Within the parameters specified above, it is possible to develop a vast number of guiding principles. Each treatment team needs to engage in discussions, and perhaps negotiations, to develop its own unique set of guiding principles. The fruits of such discussions are invaluable, enabling the treatment team to provide an orchestrated approach to working with clients. It should be possible to deal effectively with splitting attempts.

DECEPTION

A difficulty encountered by most mental health professionals working with juvenile sex offenders is a lack of knowledge and effective strategies for dealing with deception. Consequently, many treatment programs fail to address deception adequately when treating the juvenile sex offender. What we do know about deception is based on personal moral teachings. We are taught that deception is bad and we should avoid it. We are taught that if we suspect someone of being deceptive, we are suspecting them of being bad. We are taught to have unconditional acceptance of our clients and to avoid judging them and especially to avoid judging them as bad. Primitive moral strictures provide little more than conflict and confusion when it comes to dealing with deceptions. Perhaps what is called for is a more rational approach to the issue of deception.

Effective treatment of the juvenile sex offender must contend with the fact that the juvenile sex offender can be deceptive when he chooses to be. Clinicians should be aware of the types of deception, the clues to deception, and strategies for defeating deception.

Deception occurs when a person misleads a target, another person, without the target's permission. There are two types of deception: concealment and fabrication. Concealment occurs when a person withholds information without saying anything false. Fabrication occurs when a person withholds true information and presents false information as if it were true. Most persons who are experienced in deception tend to use concealment because it is simpler than fabrication. Still, it is possible to move an individual from concealment deception to fabrication deception by careful questioning. This is what occurs in law enforcement settings when a peace officer interrogates a suspect.

Ekman (1985) has identified some fundamental characteristics of deception:

1. Most deceptive people can deceive most of their targets most of the time.
2. As a person engages in deception about a particular issue, the person must also be deceptive about feelings associated with the deception (e.g., guilt).
3. Most deception is verbal because words are easy to monitor and falsify.
4. Clues to deception that are well known (e.g., poor eye contact) can easily be manipulated by a deceptive person.

5. Any emotion can be fabricated to conceal another emotion. The smile is the most commonly used mask.
6. The deceptive person censors the behavior that he expects others will watch. Words are the most commonly censored.
7. There is no certain or infallible sign of deceit. There are only signs that a person is poorly prepared or that an emotion does not fit the person's verbalization.

It is important to note the last item: There is no single clue to deceit. Some clinicians would have us believe that there are reliable means for detecting deception. As Ekman points out, this is not the case. If it were possible to reliably and consistently detect deception, the technique would be taught and we could rid the world of deception. The result would be no more criminals, car salesmen, or politicians. But there are only indirect signs of deception and these signs are cues of self-betrayal of the poorly prepared deceptive person.

Ekman suggests that there are two types of clues to deceit: leakage and cues. Leakage occurs when the person inadvertently tells the truth. Cues are signs that the person is ill-prepared to be deceptive. Table 6–1 summarizes Ekman's scheme.

It is important to note that there is more than one clue that a person is being deceitful. In fairness to the other person, several of these clues should exist before suspicion is aroused. However, if there is good reason to believe that deception exists, then the clinician should pursue the deception in an effort to uncover the truth.

A strategy known as validity interviewing can be used when a client is suspected of being deceptive. In this approach, the clinician attempts to uncover concealed information by following a four-step process:

1. *Free narrative* — The clinician allows the client to talk freely and openly. The clinician does not question but

Table 6–1.
Clues to Deceit

	Leakage	*Cues*
Speech	Slips of the tongue Tirades	Appears unprepared Hesitation Inconsistency
Voice		Pauses Inappropriate pitch

Body	Inappropriate gesture,
	  e.g., shakes head no
	  when says yes
		Decreased gesture

Face		Inappropriate expression Squelched expression Poorly timed expression

merely listens. The clinician gives supportive feedback in an effort to get the client to be expansive.

2. *Direct examination* — The clinician asks direct questions of the client. Confrontation is avoided. The clinician especially avoids asking questions about inconsistencies. The goal is to elicit additional information and fill in gaps in the client's statement.

3. *Motivational monologue* — At this point in the interview, the clinician engages in an extensive monologue designed to motivate the client to be honest. There are four things that the clinician does during this monologue:

   A. *Create reciprocity* — create a sense of camaraderie and cooperation. Emphasize the common ground between the client and the counselor.

   B. *Create a sense of urgency* — let the client know that you know information is being concealed. Explain that the costs associated with concealing information increase with time. Suggest that there is no good solution but that honesty is the least unpleasant.

     C. *Provide reasons* — suggest some reasons why the client may want to divulge the information; persuade the client that deception is not in his interest.

     D. *Ask* — ask for the desired information. If the client does divulge some information, be aware that telling a partial truth is common. Probe and attempt to uncover additional information.

4. *Cross-examination* — If the client does not reveal the concealed information, then the clinician cross-examines the client. This is the point at which the clinician confronts the client with all the inconsistencies in the client's story. It is best to confront with several inconsistencies at once so as to defeat the client's attempt to justify or minimize. The cross-examination also entails periodically returning to the motivational monologue in an attempt to further induce the client to cease the deception.

The validity-interviewing technique is based on a rational approach to dealing with deception. This approach is not intended to shame or denigrate the client in any manner. When the validity interview is done correctly, it can help the client relinquish his deception in favor of a healthy, honest stance.

Overall, it must be recognized that the juvenile sex-offending client will be deceptive. As suggested earlier, most of the time the client will succeed in the deception. When deception is detected and it is necessary to confront it, the validity interview provides for a humane, effective intervention.

PLOYS AND GAMES

The juvenile sex offender uses deception for more than just concealment. Deception can be used by the juvenile sex offender for revenge, entertainment, or establishing position in the pecking order, that is, the informal hierarchy of peers. When deception is used to meet these needs it becomes more than deception. It becomes manipulation and exploitation.

Just as there may be implicit moral strictures that prevent us from being willing to admit our clients are deceptive, impediments also exist that prevent us from calling our clients manipulative or exploitive. Yet the juvenile sex offender is exploitive and it will not do the clinician or the client any good to dress up the offender's behavior and dub it "acting out," "incompletely abreacted psychical trauma," or "unconscious conflict." The juvenile sex offender exploits others, and when the offender becomes a client he tries to exploit staff and peers. It is not a question of whether or not these clients will try to exploit others. It is a question of how much and in what manner will the client be exploitive.

In dealing with the exploitive behavior of these clients, one must recognize that they are capable of nonsexual exploitive acts as well as sexual exploitation. The juvenile sex-offending client may be manipulative regarding privileges, treatment, recreation, and a host of other nonsexual activities. Yet it is important to recognize that the juvenile sex offender will also behave in a sexually exploitive manner, for example, secretive sexual contact with peers or rape of a staff member. So, the members of the treatment team must remain alert to all forms of manipulation—sexual and nonsexual.

Perhaps it is a function of the setting, but it would appear that some of the ways in which juvenile sex-offending clients try to manipulate are consistent and to some extent predictable. Here are some of the more predictable, if not routine, ploys and games used by these clients to manipulate peers and staff:

"I'll Scratch Your Back, You Scratch Mine"

This is a ploy that is typically used by the client to manipulate other clients. In this ploy, a client may promise a peer certain favors or rewards if the peer does a certain thing. The most common bribe is designed to attain some form of sexual contact: the client promises a reward if the peer will engage in sexual contact with him. The more restrictive the environment, the more likely bribes will be used. Things that can be used as bribes include food, clothing, stereos, books, and writing supplies.

No Place Like Home

This ploy is used with a client's peer group. It entails creating a delinquent subculture that is secret and out of the awareness of the treatment team. The client begins by seeking the support of his peers for negative behavior. Rebellious behavior is deemed to be valuable and conformity to program rules is demeaned. Initially, the client avoids prosocial peers and concentrates on gaining the support of delinquent peers. After the hierarchy and social framework have been established among the delinquent peers, they begin to actively pressure and recruit the more positive peers. Little by little, staff may notice an increasingly negative atmosphere. Then, sporadic acting out will occur among clients. By the time staff recognizes that a vibrant delinquent subculture exists, it is well established. The delinquent subculture has become a home away from home.

Puppets on a String

This game entails the client convincing a peer to do something negative. The client who uses this ploy is usually a leader among his peers and has little difficulty getting weaker peers to do his "dirty work." Oftentimes, a client uses this ploy to strike out at someone without being the one who carries out the action. For example, a manipulative client may convince a weak peer that another client is going to harm him. The manipulator incites the weak peer to assault the other peer, thus accomplishing the manipulative goal of revenge.

It should be noted that sometimes a client pulls strings just to feel powerful. The client may enjoy disrupting a program or frustrating staff. The enjoyment is amplified when the manipulator does not get caught because he has gotten his peers to do the acting out.

"What Did You Expect — I'm Sick"

This ploy is usually directed at staff. In this ploy, the client hides behind his diagnosis in an effort to escape accountability for misconduct. The client typically uses the excuse of confusion or claims that what he did is not what he intended to do. If these initial rationalizations are not effective in convincing staff, then the client will claim that he lacks the skills to avoid acting out, or has not undergone the part of the treatment program that would enable him to do so. Overall, the ploy is based on the notion that the client is helpless and should not be held accountable for misconduct.

"The Sky Is Falling"

Most residential programs run on a tight schedule with rules and regulations. If staff successfully adheres to the scheduled activities, there is little opportunity for the clients to act out. Therefore, clients have learned to create deviations in a schedule by creating crises. In its most subtle and least disruptive form, a distraction can be created when one client occupies staff with a simple request, for example, "I need toothpaste," while his peers go into a restricted area or engage in a restricted activity. Not all distractions are so benign. Some clients have been known to incite fights, start a riot, or set a fire to create a distraction. While staff rallies to contend with the crisis, the client is free to engage in misconduct (e.g., escape). When dealing with a crisis, the prudent staff will keep one eye on the crisis and one eye on the clients.

Emotional Counterattack

This is a ploy that clients typically use with staff. It can be an unconscious reaction, but more commonly it is conscious and deliberate. This ploy entails engendering strong emotions in the staff, most commonly anger. Anger can be created any number of ways including engaging in rebellious behavior, verbal discussion, or threats. The more practiced client may even use information about a staff member, or his/her family, to create anger. More than anything else the client hopes that the staff person will act out his/her anger. The client will use this to justify his own anger and acting out. Some clients can even use this to influence other clients and have them believe the staff is not to be trusted. Even if the staff member does not act out, creating anger is an effective ploy. Clients know that adults cannot think straight when emotionally aroused.

"You Are the Best Staff Member"

This ploy is used by a client to split a staff member from the treatment team. Two variations on this ploy are "No one else understands me," and "I'll tell you but don't tell anyone else." All of these ploys are designed to seduce the staff member into thinking he/she has an exclusive relationship with the client. In fact, the intended relationship is not so much exclusive as it is excluding. That is, the client hopes to exclude all other staff from his treatment and only deal with one staff member. The payoff is simple: it is easier to manipulate one person than a group. Most experienced staff members know to avoid special, or exclusive, relationships with clients. Typically it is the novice or the narcissistic staff member who succumbs to this ploy.

There are many other ploys that can be used by juvenile sex-offending clients. In fact, the variety of ploys that a client could potentially use is limited only by the client's imagination and delinquent strivings. In the course of treatment, it is expected that the client's delinquent strivings will be diminished and there will be a concomitant decrease in manipulative ploys.

TREATMENT CONTRACT

It is one matter to know of potential deception and manipulation. It is another to develop a formal, programmatic response to these problems. Based upon the foregoing discussion, it is evident that the proactive treatment team will expect the juvenile sex-offending client to engage in deception and manipulation. In formulating a response to the problems, the goal is to diminish the opportunity for these problems to occur and provide a forum in which to address these problems when detected.

Perhaps the most effective mechanism for bringing manipulation and deception into the treatment arena is to develop a treatment contract. The treatment contract is a written agreement between the client and the treatment team (see client workbooks). The contract delineates the various ways in which the client may attempt to manipulate or deceive. Then, the client signs a pact with the treatment team to avoid these behaviors. Of course, the client has made many commitments in the past and he is expected to adhere to the treatment contract with the same degree of success as in the past, that is, he will be expected not to adhere to the contract. However, when he does not adhere to the contract, his deceptive and manipulative ploys become grist for the therapeutic mill and that is the importance of the treatment contract.

Previous treatment experience with juvenile sex offenders suggests certain issues should be addressed in a treatment contract. The following general categories should be included in a treatment contract:

Victims

The clients should agree to have no contact with any person whom they have previously victimized, unless such contact is supervised or controlled by the treatment team. In the event that the victim is a family member, contact with all family members should occur only in family therapy. The clients should also agree to avoid situations that could promote sexual exploitation of others (e.g., "I will never be alone with someone who is younger, smaller, or weaker than me"). It is useful to include statements in the treatment contract that address the grooming process (e.g., "I will not give gifts to peers," "I will not get a person angry or guilty so they will have sex with me").

Control of Deviant Outlets

As shown by the research, most sex offenders engage in more than one form of deviant sexual behavior. It is common for most juvenile sex offenders to have three or four behavioral outlets for their deviant sexual strivings. Therefore, the treatment contract should require the client to refrain from all types of deviant behavior (e.g., "I will not watch peers coming and going to the showers," "I will not look down the shirts or blouses of peers or staff"). One of the more common deviant sexual outlets is pornography, which should also be curtailed (e.g., "I will not have pictures of my victim," "I will not possess or put on the wall pictures of women in bathing suits, underwear, or in any state of full or partial nudity").

Therapeutic Activities

One of the main methods of manipulation entails violation of rules, guidelines, and schedules of treatment. Clients should agree to follow program rules and schedules. To the extent possible, clients should be required to inform staff when schedule conflicts arise. Clients will test limits so it is important to clearly delineate expectations so that when limit testing occurs it can be addressed in a formal treatment setting.

Confidentiality

The issue of confidentiality is frequently used in manipulative ploys by clients. The client may refuse to talk because he fears other clients at the facility may learn of his sexual misconduct. This ploy can be dealt with more easily if clients sign a treatment contract that requires them to maintain confidentiality. Another aspect of confidentiality often manipulated by clients is staff–client confidentiality. The client may promise to tell a specific staff member something critical, if that staff member will keep the information confidential. This is little more than splitting, and this behavior should be addressed in the treatment contract (e.g., "I understand that there are not secrets among staff: what I tell one staff, I tell all").

The more detailed and simple the treatment contract, the more effective it will be. It is recommended that the treatment contract be divided into the categories listed above. Within each category, items should be listed in a simple straightforward manner. When possible a treatment item should be one sentence, or at most two sentences. The treatment contract is not used to control clients; it is used to bring the client's manipulative and deceptive behavior into the formal treatment arena.

CONCLUSIONS

With all this attention given to countertransference, deception, and manipulation, readers are likely to have one of two reactions. On the one hand, readers might feel discouraged and wonder if they are in the right field. If that is your reaction, then you need to consider that you may be better suited to deal with some other clientele. On the other hand, some readers may feel confident that they have the tools to avoid ever being manipulated by these clients. If that is your reaction, then you are most certainly in the wrong field, or, at a minimum, you have misunderstood this chapter.

It is a fact: these clients stir primitive, visceral emotions in the clinician. It is a fact: these clients are frequently manipulative and deceptive. The clinician must recognize and accept these facts if treatment is to be effective. The clinician who cannot accept these facts should consider working with some other clientele.

Where does the satisfaction come from when working with these clients? Ideally, the satisfaction should come from oneself. The clinician capable of intrinsic reward is the one best suited for work with this population. Intrinsic reward is the reward that people give themselves for a job well done. It is possible to intervene effectively with the juvenile sex offender. It is possible to reduce the likelihood that these clients will re-offend. While this should be encouraging to those working with this clientele, it should be recognized that the real satisfaction should come from within.

APPENDIX A

**The Bridges Program
Client Workbook**

CONTENTS

INTRODUCTION

This is the workbook that you will use in therapy. All of the things that you must do in therapy are in this workbook.

Things are put into this workbook to help you be different. The most important thing is you must be different with people. You must not hurt people. You cannot use sex or anything else to hurt people. This workbook will help you make sure that you don't hurt other people.

You probably have done lots of schoolwork and homework. You know this type of work can be hard. The work in this book is important but it is not supposed to be hard. You will have the chance to make up your own games, posters, and songs. A lot of the things in this book will be fun.

One last thing to remember about this book: share what you learn. If you learn something new, talk to your friends about it. Tell staff members about it. Tell your family. The more you share, the better you become.

BINDING AGREEMENTS

Stages of Treatment

Prestage: Orientation

Tasks:

_____ 1. Complete the orientation program.
_____ 2. Complete the orientation quiz.
_____ 3. Complete the truth worksheet.
_____ 4. Present the truth worksheet to staff.
_____ 5. Present the truth worksheet to parents.
_____ 6. Present the truth worksheet in group.

Goals:

_____ 1. Learn about the program.
_____ 2. Understand how to give and receive help.
_____ 3. Begin to be open about sex deviance.

Stage One: Concept Formation

Tasks:

_____ 1. Positive and deviant sex pictures
_____ 2. Offense cycle poster/handout
_____ 3. Victim story role plan
_____ 4. Clarification letter
_____ 5. Stay away, look away, get away worksheet
_____ 6. Complete fourteen (14) positive attitude worksheets.

Gcals:

_____ 1. Learn the difference between positive and deviant sex.
_____ 2. Be able to stop offense cycle in group.

_____ 3. Be able to give and receive help in group.

_____ 4. Be able to recognize harm done to others in group.

_____ 5. Be able to stop self from acting out in group.

_____ 6. Be able to recognize thinking errors in group.

Stage Two: Transfer of Training

Tasks:

_____ 1. Sexual development book report

_____ 2. Offense Cycle game

_____ 3. Empathy homework

_____ 4. Role play "The Gifts"

_____ 5. Temptation song

_____ 6. Thinking Error homework

Goals:

_____ 1. Use appropriate touch in group and on campus.

_____ 2. Be able to stop cycle when not in group.

_____ 3. Be able to stop hurting others.

_____ 4. Be able to give help in and out of group.

_____ 5. Avoid or escape acting out.

_____ 6. Be able to self-correct thinking errors.

Stage Three: Generalization and Practice

Tasks:

_____ 1. Role play discussion of healthy sex.

_____ 2. Offense Cycle lesson plan

_____ 3. Presentation of clarification letter

_____ 4. Empathy Care game

_____ 5. Relapse Prevention plan

_____ 6. Smart-Talk poster

Goals:

_____ 1. Confront others who use inappropriate touch.
_____ 2. Stop own cycle and confront others in cycle.
_____ 3. Be able to express empathy.
_____ 4. Be able to give and receive help.
_____ 5. Set a positive example for peers.
_____ 6. Be able to correct own thinking errors.

Stage Four: Transition Planning

Tasks:

_____ 1. Complete personal schedule.
_____ 2. Complete transition plan.
_____ 3. Share relapse prevention plan with outpatient therapist.

Goals:

_____ 1. Prepare for transition to the community.
_____ 2. Begin transferring skills and learning to new situations.

Treatment Contract

I. *Victims*
A. *Non-Incest Victims*
1. I will not talk to, write, telephone, or contact my victim.
2. I will not respond if my victim tries to contact me.
3. I will not send messages to my victim through other people.
4. I will not send gifts to my victim.
5. I will not make requests of my victim.
6. I will have contact with my victim only when my Sexual Treatment Services therapist says it is appropriate.
B. *Incest Victims*
1. All rules listed in I. A (1–6) apply.
2. I will not participate in family therapy with my victim until I have completed clarification.
3. I will not have an on-campus or off-campus visit with my family if my victim accompanies my family, unless I have completed clarification.
4. I will not visit home until I complete clarification.
C. *Potential Victims*
1. I will never be alone with someone who is younger, smaller, or weaker than me.
2. I will never be alone with someone who is physically or mentally handicapped.
3. I will be escorted by staff everywhere I go until I earn the privilege of being unsupervised.
4. I will not go to the bathroom if someone else is there.

5. I will not tell secrets or gossip with peers.
6. I will not work in jobs that require me to be alone with peers or have limited supervision around peers.
7. I will not give gifts to peers, unless approved by my Sexual Treatment Services therapist.
8. I will not force a person to have sex with me.
9. I will not trick, bribe, or groom a person to have sex with me.
10. I will not get a person angry, guilty, or sad so that they will have sex with me.
11. I will not have sexual contact with a person who has been drinking alcohol or using drugs.
12. I will not have sexual contact with anyone under the age of legal consent.
13. I will not undress where other people can observe me.

II. *Control of Deviant Outlets*
1. I will not buy or possess pornography.
2. I will not display pictures in my personal space that could be considered sexual, e.g., bathing suit ads, some rock 'n' roll posters, underwear commercials, etc. My Sexual Treatment Services therapist will determine if pictures are appropriate for display.
3. I will not watch peers coming and going to the showers. I will not watch peers in the shower.
4. I will not look at peers or staff in a sexual manner.
5. I will not talk with peers in the dorm about sexual matters.

6. I will not eavesdrop on peers or staff.
7. I will not touch people without permission.
8. I will not use animals in sexual acts.
9. I will not masturbate to deviant fantasies.
10. I will not walk or ride about aimlessly so as to watch for potential victims.
11. I will not scout areas or set up situations for sexual acting out.
12. I will not go to movies or get books, videos, or magazines that contain sexual scenes or material.
13. I will not look down the blouses of women, girls, or other victims.
14. I will not rate other persons in terms of the presence or absence of sexual appeal.
15. I will not stare at the sexual body parts of other persons.
16. I will not discuss sexual fantasies about other persons outside of group or individual therapy.
17. I will not make sexual gestures or moon others.

III. *Therapeutic Activities*

1. I will attend all therapy activities in the Sexual Treatment Services.
2. I will be on time for all Sexual Treatment Services activities.
3. I will comply with the Group Rules, Treatment Contract, and Stages of Treatment.
4. I will complete all homework assignments by the deadlines set by the Sexual Treatment Services therapist.
5. I will be responsible for informing other staff of my appointments with Sexual Treatment Services.
6. I will not allow other activities or passes to

interfere with my Sexual Treatment Services appointments.
7. I will get permission from my Sexual
   Treatment Services therapist for exceptions
   to items 1-6.
8. I will talk about sexual matters only in
   group therapies or individual therapies.

IV. *Confidentiality*
1. I understand that there are no secrets
   among treatment staff. What I tell one staff,
   I tell all.
2. I understand that staff will talk to my
   victim's therapist about what is said in
   treatment.
3. I understand that staff will talk to my
   insurance company about my treatment.
4. If I am on probation, parole, court order, or
   state mandate, I understand that staff will
   talk to the appropriate persons in the legal
   system.
5. I understand that staff will talk to others to
   stop me if I harm or threaten to harm
   myself or anyone else.
6. I understand that staff must report to the
   state any victim who is a minor, elderly, or
   disabled.
7. I understand that staff may permit visitors
   to observe some therapy sessions.

_____   _____
Client   Date

_____   _____
Sexual Treatment   Date
Services Therapist

Group Rules

Grooming

- Be free of body odor.
- Have your hair combed.
- Dress neatly.
- Do not wear hats or sunglasses in group.

During Group

- Pay attention.
- Listen to others.
- Keep your chair on the ground.
- Keep seated.
- Give help.
- Receive help.
- Be honest.
- Use people's names (not *dude, homeboy, hey you*).

Between Groups

- Do all homework.
- Do not talk to others about group.
- Follow all treatment guidelines.

I understand and agree to follow these rules.

_____   _____
Client   Date

_____   _____
Sexual Treatment   Date
Services Therapist

ORIENTATION

Therapy Goals

Therapy is when two or more people talk and try to solve problems. In this program, therapy will happen lots of different ways.

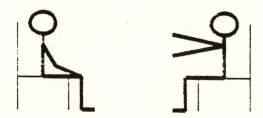

You may have individual therapy. This is when you meet with just one other person, a therapist.

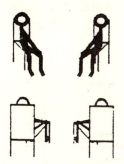

You will also have family therapy. This is when you meet with your family and at least one therapist. The most important therapy that you will have is group therapy. This is when you meet with a therapist and several peers who have the same problem that you have.

No matter what type of therapy you are doing, the goal of this program is always the same. Your goal in therapy is to never hurt another person, and especially to never hurt another person by using sex. If you reach this goal, your life will be better because you will not get into trouble. Also other people, including your family, will be happier and safer if you reach your goal. Remember, the goal of treatment is: No More Victims.

How Change Happens

Life is full of change. Some changes are good. Other changes are bad. This program helps you make good changes. It takes at least three steps to change a behavior. They are:

1. Be self-aware. You must be able to look at yourself, like looking into a mirror. You must be able to see how your actions hurt you and others. When you see how you hurt others you will want to change.

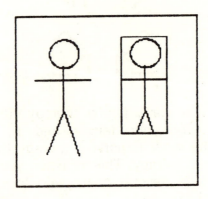

2. Self-monitor. You must learn to see the signs that you are heading down the path of harmful behavior. You must learn the signs that tell you that you are about to do wrong.

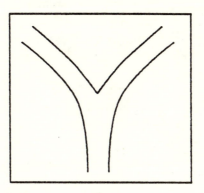

3. Self-control. You must learn how to be your own boss. You have to be powerful. You must use your power to control yourself.

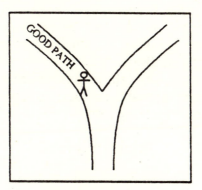

Thinking Errors

Thinking determines feelings and actions.

Events don't cause feelings; thoughts cause feelings. Between every event and feeling, there is a thought.

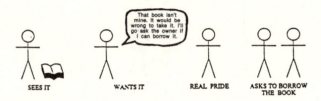

Event → Thinking → Feeling → Action

Even when an event stays the same, if a person's thinking changes, the feeling and actions will change.

Some thinking is true and leads to honest, caring actions; other thinking is untrue and leads to dishonest, hurtful actions. You will learn the thinking errors and smart self-talk in positive-attitudes group. Thinking errors sometimes lead to deviant sex. We will talk about thinking errors in this group.

Thinking Errors

Feel It, Do It: This is when people think that their emotions caused their thoughts or actions.

Alternative smart self-talk: Recognize that your thoughts cause your feelings and actions.

Poor Me: This is when you try to get others to feel sorry for you to avoid responsibility for your actions.

Alternative smart self-talk: Accept your part and your responsibility in a situation before focusing on the other person's part in a situation.

I Can't: This is when you say you cannot do something as an excuse for not really trying to do it.

Alternative smart self-talk: Try to do something whether it is exciting or not.

Mindreading: This is when you assume you know what others are thinking without asking.

Alternative smart self-talk: Ask.

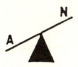

All or Nothing: This is when you say things like: "Everyone does it" or "This never happens." Other "All or Nothing" words are: Nobody, All, None, Now, Never, Always, Everything, Nothing.

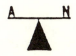

Alternative smart self-talk: Think about life as a series of steps or a balance between two things.

Urges and Fantasies

Before a person can do any action, the person must think about the action. Actions do not just happen. People think before they act.

Before a person uses deviant sex, the person must think about the deviant sex. There are two ways a person can think about sex:

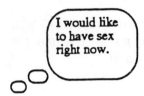

Urge—a person has an urge when the person has thoughts or feelings after they look at another person in a sexual way. For example, if a boy looks at a girl and says, "She is pretty," that is an urge. An urge can be either deviant or positive.

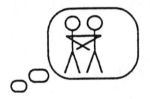

Fantasy—a fantasy is the picture in your mind. If you see yourself touching the person, kissing the person, or holding the person, you are having a fantasy.

Urges and fantasies always come before a sex act. You cannot have a sex act without first thinking about it.

Urge → Fantasy → Act

If a person has deviant urges, then deviant fantasies will occur. If the person has a deviant fantasy, then a deviant act will occur.

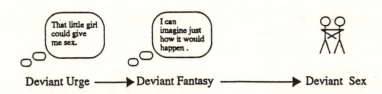

Deviant Urge ⟶ Deviant Fantasy ⟶ Deviant Sex

If a person wants to stop deviant sex, the solution is easy: replace deviant thinking with thoughts about positive sex.

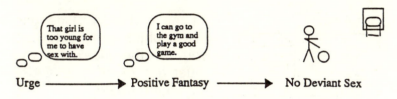

Urge ⟶ Positive Fantasy ⟶ No Deviant Sex

Stay Away, Look Away, Get Away

A high-risk situation can be people, places, or things that remind you of deviant sex. A park is a high-risk place because children play there. A child is a high-risk person. A high-risk thing is pornography because it can cause sexual urges. Alcohol is a high-risk thing because it can lead to bad decisions about sex. A high-risk situation tempts you to have deviant sexual urges or deviant sexual fantasies.

There are at least three things you can do to handle high-risk people, high-risk places, and high-risk things:

Stay Away:

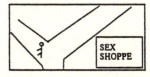

Stay away from people, places, or things that put you in danger. Can you think of any situation you should stay away from?

Look Away:

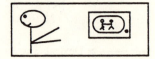

Sometimes you will find yourself around children or other high-risk situations. Always think of something else. Leave as soon as you can. Look away until you can leave. How would you cope with children on a bus?

Get Away:

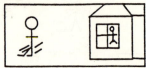

At the first sign of danger, like a child walking toward you on the sidewalk, you must get away ... ESCAPE ... Right away!

Giving and Receiving Help

There are only two things that a client can do in therapy. A client can either Give Help or Receive Help. A client Gives Help by doing any of the following:

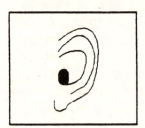

- Pay attention and listen to the therapists or group members.
- Give support to a group member who feels bad.
- Confront a group member who is acting mean, rude, or deviant.

A client Receives Help by doing any of the following:

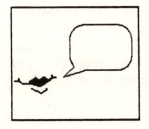

- Pay attention to therapists and other group members when they talk.
- Learn how other persons' situations apply to you.
- Do not argue when other people give you feedback.

There is only one way to get better. A person must go to therapy. But going to therapy is not enough. While in therapy, the person must give help and receive help. Before you say anything or do anything in therapy, ask yourself this question: "Does that give or receive help?"

Group Therapy

In this program, group therapy is very important. You will be in group therapy sessions with peers who share your problems and issues. The goal of therapy is to eliminate deviant sex so that there are No More Victims. You can reach this goal, and help your peers reach this goal, by giving help and receiving help.

The way group therapy is done in this program is a little different from the usual group therapy. There are very specific and special ways that a group works. This is how a group is run:

Beginning—Each group begins with group members doing a layout. A layout is when people talk about themselves and pick a topic to discuss.

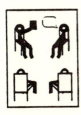

Middle—This is when group members give help and receive help. Group members can talk about tasks or worksheets they have done or need to do.

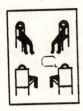

End—The session comes to an end. The group therapist tells you how you did during the session.

As you can see, there is only one way to do group. To be successful, each person must be able to pick a problem to work on every session. When you are not working on your own problems, you need to help peers work on their problems.

Sex Words

In this therapy, we will be talking a great deal about sex. People have many words for talking about sex. In therapy, we only use words that show respect for others. Street language and slang words are not okay. Here is a list of words to use.

Male Body
penis
scrotum
testicles
rectum
anus
buttocks

Female Body
breasts
vagina
ovaries
rectum
anus
buttocks

Deviant Sex
  Behavior
rape
child molest
touch without permission
expose
peep
fetish
theft

Positive Sex
  Behavior
kiss
fondle
intercourse
hug
hold hands

PRESTAGE: ORIENTATION

Truth Worksheet

I am in sex offender treatment because _____
_____
_____ .

The last time I sexually abused someone was
_____ when I _____
_____
_____ .

I set up my victims by _____
_____
_____ .

It's easier for me to sexually abuse others when
_____
_____ .

Others can help me avoid sexually abusing people
by _____
_____
_____ .

Areas where I might re-offend here are _____
_____
_____ .

Orientation Quiz

1. One example of "Giving Help" in group is: _____

_____

_____

_____

_____ .

2. One example of "Receiving Help" in group is: _

_____

_____

_____

_____ .

3. My treatment contract includes things I will do:
   a. in group only
   b. everywhere

4. If I complete the tasks of the group and practice new behaviors I will meet the goals of the group.

   TRUE or FALSE

5. My group therapist promises that I will never sexually abuse again if I complete all tasks and goals of this program.

   TRUE or FALSE

STAGE ONE: CONCEPT FORMATION

Layout

My name is _____ .

My offense was _____ .

My victim(s)' name(s): _____

My cycle of abuse includes hurting myself and others by _____

_____ .

I have broken my treatment contract this week by

_____ .

I have had _____ deviant urges or fantasies this week.

I stopped them by _____ .

The task I want to complete today is _____

_____ .

Deviant and Positive Sex

There are two ways to have sex. One way to have sex is bad. It hurts people. This is called Deviant Sex. The other way to have sex is good. Positive Sex does not hurt other people. The definition for positive sex is presented below:

Positive sex is:

1. Sex between two people who love each other and who are not close relatives.

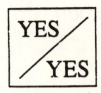

2. Each time the two people have sex, both agree to have sex.

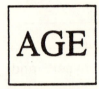

3. Sex with someone old enough to legally agree.

4. Sex that doesn't include force or tricks, yelling, bribes, threats, money, shame, or fear.

Sometimes people use deviant sex. Deviant sex is always wrong. It is the opposite of positive sex. It is not loving. Deviant sex is between two people who don't agree to have sex. It involves force. It is sex between two people who can't legally agree to have sex (relatives/minors). People who use deviant sex can learn to use positive sex. Positive sex is good. People should use only positive sex.

Offense Cycle Handout

Cut out the cards along the dotted lines and use the cards while describing your own cycle of offending.

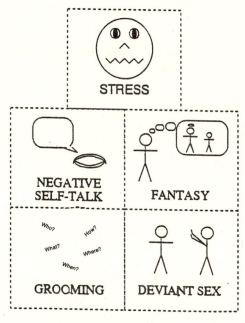

STRESS

NEGATIVE SELF-TALK

FANTASY

Who? How? What? Where? When?

GROOMING

DEVIANT SEX

Victim's Story

For each victim you sexually abused, ask for time in group to tell how each victim might describe his/her abuse. Tell what the victim might have thought before, during, and after the abuse happened. If you abused a victim more than one time, tell how the victim would describe the first time or the last time. When you are done, answer questions from group members. Remember, your victim probably answered a lot of questions from parents, teachers, police officers, and others.

Clarification Letter

Dear _____ ,

I am writing today to _____ .

In this letter I will _____ .

I will answer any other questions you have also. If you give me permission I will continue this letter. I chose you as my victim because I noticed these good things about you: _____ .

I used thinking errors to change my thinking about your good qualities. I made myself think _____ about you.

You did not cause the abuse to happen. I did. I set up the abuse by _____ .

Before I abused you I controlled you by _____ .

I hid my bad plans by _____ .

I misused your trust. It was normal for you to trust me when I falsely acted like _____ .

I sexually abused you by _____ in the beginning. Then I _____ . At the end I _____ .

You said _____ . I continued to control you and be dishonest by _____ .

In order to make you keep it a secret I _____ .

You did many things to stop me. You _____
_____ .
I knew you were being hurt because _____
_____
_____ .
I believe you may be hurt in other ways now such
as _____
_____
_____
_____ .
I believe my abusive behavior also hurt others
including _____
_____
_____ .
It was my responsibility to not _____
_____ to you. It is all my fault.
I would like to ask _____ if _____ can carry the
feelings of _____, _____, about the
sexual abuse because it was _____ fault. In
treatment I have learned that positive sex is
different from deviant sex. Deviant sex is _____
_____ . Positive sex is _____
_____ .
It is _____ responsibility to never use deviant
sex again. I misused your feelings of safety in the
world by _____ .
I hope you will feel safe again around me because
_____
_____
_____ .
I will be responsible for doing things to only make
you feel safe around me. I will _____
_____
_____ .

Sincerely,

_____
_____ (date)

Stay Away, Look Away, Get Away Worksheet

Complete as many of these as your group therapist recommends. You may complete them for high-risk situations at this facility or for off-campus outings. After reading the handout, fill in how you will Stay Away, Look Away, and Get Away from five possible temptations of deviant sex in the situation you are currently preparing for.

Temptation:

1. _____
   Stay Away _____
   Look Away _____
   Get Away _____
2. _____
   Stay Away _____
   Look Away _____
   Get Away _____
3. _____
   Stay Away _____
   Look Away _____
   Get Away _____
4. _____
   Stay Away _____
   Look Away _____
   Get Away _____
5. _____
   Stay Away _____
   Look Away _____
   Get Away _____

Positive Attitude Worksheet

---

1. Name   2. Date

---

3. Problem Behavior:

---

4. Thinking Error I used:

---

5. Smart Self-Talk I could have used:

---

6. Three past/future situations that might prove smart self-talk is true:

1.   2.

3.

STAGE TWO: TRANSFER OF TRAINING

Book Report

I read/listened to the story called _____
_____ .
_____ in the story was doing things that are positive sex. The cues of positive sex were _____
_____
_____ .
_____ in the story was doing things that are deviant sex. The cues of deviant sex were _____
_____
_____ .
My past life is a little like _____ in the story because we both _____
_____ .
If I could give advice to _____ in the story about his/her deviant sex I would tell him/her ____
_____
_____ .
If I could support _____ for using positive sex I would tell him/her _____
_____ .
One new thing this story made me think about is _____ .

Cycle Game

Pick a type of game you know well and can teach others, for example, a card game, a board game, or an action game.

Tell the group and your therapist what materials you will need to create a game that teaches others about the five steps in the offense cycle.

Make the game and explain it to the group.

Play the game with the group.

Discuss how it felt to teach something new to others.

Discuss how it will feel to discuss what you are learning in group with others in your life who might need to know.

Empathy Homework

I encouraged the following peers to think about their behavior and to not hurt others. Staff signed when they heard me do this:

Peer's initials   Date   Staff signature

1.

2.

3.

4.

5.

6.

7.

"The Gifts"

One day a teenage boy was walking down the street feeling bored. The boy was walking along kicking a can until he spotted another person walking toward him. From far away the boy noticed how he and the stranger had things in common. The other person was relaxed and not in a hurry. The other person seemed to enjoy kicking a can along, too. Then the boy noticed the person's shoes, which he didn't like at all. A few seconds later he began focusing on himself. He began feeling anger about how his parents refused to let him borrow the car last night. They said he had to do chores around the house to earn gas money. This boy didn't want to do homework and chores every night. He decided his parents were unfair. As he walked and kept thinking these thoughts about only himself, something happened. When he looked up, the other person walking down the street no longer seemed like a whole person. All the boy saw walking toward him was two legs and two hands holding a bunch of gift boxes. As the boy got closer he thought about the sparkling packages. The boy thought that stealing those gifts would make him feel better now. He thought it would be "OK" by focusing on the shoes the person was wearing. He decided that anyone wearing such awful shoes didn't deserve gifts anyway. The boy walked closer and tried to take the gifts away. He was able to knock some of the gifts out of the person's hands and damaged some of the boxes before running away. The boy noticed that it was his father coming with the gifts. The boy felt bad after seeing the damage that was done and promised never to do it again. He vowed always to remember that whenever feeling selfish or thinking selfish thoughts, he might not be seeing the whole person behind the gifts. He vowed to remember that there is never a reason to steal another's gifts, even if you don't like something about the person, like their *shoes.*

"GIFTS" WORKSHEET

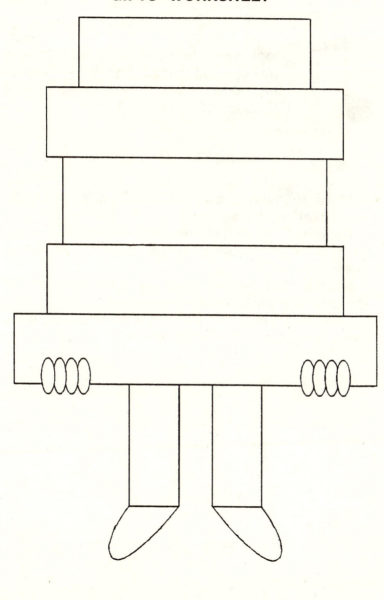

Temptation Song

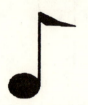

Write a song about how to stay away, look away, and get away from people, places, and things that tempt you to have deviant sex. Write it to the tune of a song most people know.

Thinking Error Homework

Make fourteen copies of the Positive Attitudes worksheet from stage one.

Complete up to two worksheets per day using your use of thinking errors outside of group sessions.

Have a staff member read and sign each one on the day you complete it.

When all fourteen worksheets are completed, bring them to group and talk about them.

STAGE THREE: GENERALIZATION AND PRACTICE

Healthy Sexual Role Play

Use a group session to role play how you will tell your family what you have learned about healthy versus deviant sex.

Use your poster or worksheet from stage one and two to teach your family.

Role play what your family members might say during this session.

Offense Cycle Lesson Plan

Role play in group how you will teach your family about your cycle.

Use materials from stages one or two to help you teach them.

Role play what questions they might have.

Empathy Card Game

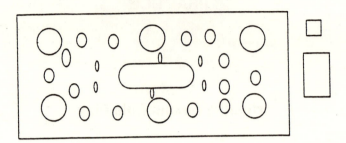

RULES OF THE GAME

1. Each player picks a colored token game piece and places it on the matching colored circle on the board.

2. Each player rolls the dice. The order of play begins with the person who first rolls a six. The order of play then goes clockwise to the left of the beginning player.

3. The first player rolls the dice again and picks a card. If the other players agree that the first player gave an appropriately empathic answer, then that first player moves to the left (clockwise) the number of spaces of the dice.

4. Next, the player to the left of the first player rolls the dice. All subsequent plays follow the directions in #3.

5. The winner is the person who circles the board and lands on his/her home space. He/she can stay there until rolling a 3, which allows him/her to move diagonally into the winner's circle.

Relapse Prevention Plan

Discuss the relapse process with your group and fill in the following steps in the relapse process as you plan for potential problems and solutions.

What if "this" happens?	(Solution) "I can/will"

Smart-Talk Poster

On a piece of large white paper (you can get this from your group therapist), glue words and pictures that represent your smart self-talk. You can glue the words of your thinking errors on it as long as you make a large *X* across the top of each word. Add pictures and words that will encourage you to use your smart self-talk.

Save this poster to use in a family therapy session. Make it look nice enough to hang in your room.

STAGE FOUR: TRANSITION PLANNING

Schedule Worksheet

When you leave this facility to go to your next placement, or home, you need to have a schedule of activities to avoid relapse. For every half hour, list what you will be doing. Schedule work and school activities first. When you list fun or play activities, list what they are and who you will be with. This schedule should be presented in one of your last groups. Revise it with the feedback you get.

	Sun	Mon	Tue	Wed	Thu	Fri	Sat
6:00–7:00							
7:00–8:00							
8:00–9:00							
9:00–10:00							
10:00–11:00							
11:00–12:00							
12:00–1:00							

and so on
to 9:00 P.M.

Transition Plan

Whenever people leave one place to go to another, it's normal to have many strong feelings about the place you are leaving and the place you are going. Sometimes old behaviors return under stress. If you plan for this you will be able to cope with whatever happens. To help you prepare to leave this program, answer the following questions to share in one of your last groups:

1. What were you like when you entered this program?

2. How have you changed? What are you like now?

3. What are the happiest, saddest, scariest, and angriest moments you had?

4. Who helped you the most? How do you feel about that person? How do you say good-bye to him/her?

5. Write a general good-bye to everyone else you've met here.

6. Describe any thoughts of nervousness you have about leaving. How can you cope with them?

7. Under stress, are you showing any signs of falling back into old behavior patterns?

8. What are they? If they continue after you leave, how will you cope?

9. Write three to five "what-ifs" about leaving here and any old behaviors that might come back. How will you handle each one?

APPENDIX B

The Renaissance Program
Client Workbook

CONTENTS

INTRODUCTION

This workbook is designed to help people with deviant sexual urges develop a more positive sexuality. It is recognized that deviant sex hurts many people including the victim and the perpetrator and all those who know or come in contact with them. Because deviant sex is so harmful, a special program has been developed to help people stop using deviant sex. Since all people are sexual, the program does not try to eliminate all sexual urges and behaviors. Rather, the main goal of the program is to replace deviant sex with positive sex so that there are no more victims.

The program that this workbook is based upon is very structured. That is, specific therapy tasks and assignments have been developed. All tasks and assignments are based upon information about what it takes to replace deviant sex with positive sex. Not only are there many tasks in the program, but these tasks are arranged in a specific order. Consider the stages of treatment of this program.

Prestage: Group Skills and Orientation

During this stage of treatment, clients are required to develop skills and knowledge that would help them succeed in group. Since clients are not expected to have knowledge or skills to be good group members, specific training is conducted to teach group skills. During this stage, clients also begin the effort to become open and honest about their deviant sex behavior.

Stage One: Cycle of Abuse
and Deviant Arousal

During this stage of treatment, clients must uncover and identify their personal pattern of sexual deviance. Once the pattern is uncovered, clients are challenged to develop coping skills to control deviant urges and eliminate deviant behavior. Some specific techniques are taught to clients that enable them to overcome deviant thoughts and fantasies.

Stage Two: Victim Empathy and Restitution

Deviant sex behavior hurts people. It is assumed that people who realize the harm caused by deviant sex won't engage in deviant sex. It is also assumed that clients in the program fail to appreciate the harm they caused to their victims. Therefore, during this stage of treatment, clients engage in therapeutic activities to increase their empathy for others. Some clients are allowed to participate in clarification, i.e., a meeting with the victim in which the client clarifies how he/she exploited the victim and why victims are not at fault for their own victimization.

Stage Three: Relapse Prevention and
Positive Arousal

Clients who are able to make it to stage three have accomplished a great deal. These clients have changed. The focus now becomes helping clients hold on to the positive changes that they have already made. This is called relapse prevention. That is, clients learn specific skills to avoid relapsing, or falling back into a pattern of deviant sexual behavior. During this stage of treatment, clients also complete assignments designed to allow them to discover positive ways of expressing their sexuality.

Stage Four: Outpatient Treatment

Clients must prepare for the transition from intensive inpatient treatment to less intense outpatient treatment. Clients are required to make specific plans for this transition. Clients are evaluated for their ability to use positive skills in a variety of settings.

The Stages of Treatment are designed to help clients become more and more positive. The first two stages just require clients to be honest and develop some self-awareness. The final stages of treatment really challenge the clients to become caring for others and exhibit self-control. While the tasks in this workbook may be difficult, the reward for accomplishing these tasks is tremendous — No More Victims.

ORIENTATION
and
TREATMENT GUIDELINES

The Orientation *section and the binding agreements for this program can be found in the Bridges Program workbook. Clients need to be aware of all binding agreements. They must agree to and sign all agreement forms prior to beginning treatment.*

Stages of Treatment

*Prestage: Group Skills
and Orientation*

Tasks

DATE   STAFF
       INITIAL

____   ____ 1. Complete Orientation sessions.
____   ____ 2. Sign treatment contract.
____   ____ 3. Complete Deviant Sex worksheet.
____   ____ 4. Deviant Sex worksheet approved in group.
____   ____ 5. Present Deviant Sex worksheet to parent/guardian.
____   ____ 6. Present Deviant Sex worksheet to core team.
____   ____ 7. Complete Orientation quiz.
____   ____ 8. Sign Group Rules contract.
____   ____ 9. Begin Skill Training.

Goals

DATE   STAFF
      INITIAL

____   ____ 1. Learn basic information about treatment.
____   ____ 2. Admit to deviant sexual behavior.
____   ____ 3. Openly accept responsibility for deviant sexual behavior.
____   ____ 4. Understand how to Give Help and Receive Help in many places.

Stage I: Cycle of Abuse and Deviant Arousal

Tasks

DATE   STAFF
        INITIAL

_____ _____ 1. Memorize Layout.

_____ _____ 2. Read Positive Sex vs. Deviant Sex, and memorize definitions.

_____ _____ 3. Complete Offense Cycle worksheet and receive group/therapist approval.

_____ _____ 4. Complete two covert sensitization worksheets.

_____ _____ 5. Begin Positive Attitude group.

_____ _____ 6. Participate in family therapy.

Goals

DATE   STAFF
        INITIAL

_____ _____ 1. Client is able to recognize abusive behavior in the offense cycle at least 75% of the time.

_____ _____ 2. Client is aware of how to get out of cycle and does this in all places at least 50% of the time.

_____ _____ 3. Client is aware of when thinking errors are being used and can switch to smart self-talk 40–60% of the time.

_____ _____ 4. Client knows what kind of fantasies are deviant and can change them to plans for positive, healthy actions at least 50% of the time.

_____ _____ 5. Client expresses fewer feelings of deprivation while actively engaging in prosocial nonsexual physical activities at least 75% of the time.

Stage II: Victim Empathy and Restitution

Tasks

DATE   STAFF
       INITIAL

____ ____ 1. Tell your victim's story to the group by role playing that you are the victim telling the story.

____ ____ 2. Complete two "40 others" worksheets and present to group.

____ ____ 3. Complete a letter of clarification to your victim.

____ ____ 4. When possible, participate in a therapy session with your victim to make restitution.

____ ____ 5. Present two more sensitization worksheets to group.

____ ____ 6. Participate in Sex Trauma group if you were sexually abused.

____ ____ 7. Participate in family therapy.

____ ____ 8. Successfully complete Positive Attitudes group requirements with 75–100% accuracy.

Goals

DATE   STAFF
       INITIAL

____ ____ 1. Appreciate the harm of sexually offending another person.

____ ____ 2. Stop harming others in any secretive or hurtful way.

____ ____ 3. Make emotional restitution to those you have hurt.

____ ____ 4. Improve your ability to break deviant arousal.

_____ _____ 5. Recognize your use of Thinking Errors and switch to Smart Self-talk.

Stage III: Relapse Prevention and Positive Arousal

Tasks

DATE   STAFF
       INITIAL

_____ _____ 1. Complete ACE worksheets.

_____ _____ 2. Role play one incident of abuse and explain how you could have used ACE to not offend.

_____ _____ 3. Complete a Relapse Prevention Plan.

_____ _____ 4. Present Relapse Prevention Plan to group.

_____ _____ 5. Present Relapse Prevention Plan to core team for approval.

_____ _____ 6. Present Relapse Prevention Plan to family.

_____ _____ 7. Discuss positive sexuality and use of power in Gender Issues group.

_____ _____ 8. Present completed Healthy Sexual Expressions worksheet to group.

_____ _____ 9. Present completed Healthy Sexual Expressions worksheet to family.

_____ _____ 10. Participate in family therapy.

_____ _____ 11. Participate in at least two assertiveness sessions on weekends.

Goals

DATE   STAFF
       INITIAL

_____ _____ 1. Appreciate the possibility of relapse—no cure.

_____ _____ 2. Be able to know high-risk situations and how to avoid, cope, or escape them without hurting self or others.

_____ _____ 3. Use a realistic plan to avoid threatening situations.

_____ _____ 4. Be able to confront others assertively using suggested format.

_____ _____ 5. Consistently express all feelings in an assertive manner to avoid relapse.

_____ _____ 6. Understand and commit to healthy sexual expression.

Stage IV: Outpatient Treatment

Tasks

DATE   STAFF
        INITIAL

_____ _____ 1. Complete a schedule for school, work, sports, and other activities to avoid stress and meet your responsibilities.

_____ _____ 2. Complete a Transition Plan and have it approved in group and by the core team.

_____ _____ 3. Attend and participate in individual group and family sessions as required.

_____ _____ 4. Complete other assignments assigned by outpatient therapist.

Goals

DATE   STAFF
        INITIAL

_____ _____ 1. Transfer skills from treatment center to the community.

_____ _____ 2. Demonstrate an ability to cope with the possibility of relapse without re-offending.

PRESTAGE: GROUP SKILLS AND ORIENTATION

Layout

My name is _____ .

My offense was _____ .

In my lifetime I have done:

____	Child Molest	____	Pornography
____	Rape	____	Frottage
____	Expose	____	Cruising
____	Peep	____	Dissecting

Since the last group session I have failed to accept responsibility for my actions _____ times.

Since the last group session I have denied that I did certain acts _____ times.

My topic for today is _____ .

Directions for Therapeutic Tasks

Orientation

Purpose: To teach new clients the skills and information they will need to succeed in the treatment program.

Description: During the Orientation, each client will typically meet individually with a therapist. The therapist will read aloud and discuss the information contained in the *Orientation* section. Patients are expected to learn, and even memorize, the information presented during orientation. There are nine lessons in the Orientation curriculum. It is likely that it will take four or more sessions to cover all this material.

Directions:

1. The client will meet with a staff person for the purpose of orientation. The staff person will schedule all appointments.
2. During these sessions, the staff person will read each lesson to the client. (Note: Orientation lessons can be found in the first section of this workbook.)
3. The staff person does not read a page to the client in its entirety. Instead, the staff person reads one paragraph at a time and explains each concept in each paragraph.
4. Staff who conduct orientation may assign homework to clients. Clients must complete all homework.

Deviant Sex Worksheet

Purpose: To help clients take an honest look at one deviant sexual act and share this information with staff and family.

Description: Deviant sex does not just happen. Something always leads up to a deviant sex act. The person who uses deviant sex may not be aware of it at the time, but if he/she reviews the act, it will become obvious that the act was planned. The purpose of this worksheet is to help each client become more honest regarding how they planned and engaged in deviant sex.

Without a doubt, denial is the obstacle that can defeat a client most easily. If a client is to complete this therapeutic task, the client must be very honest. The client cannot deny his/her role in the deviant sexual behavior.

Most people think denial occurs when a person does not admit to a deviant sex act. There is more to denial than this. A deviant sex act has a beginning, middle, and end. Therefore, denial can occur at all three of these phases of a deviant sex act. Consider this:

Phase	Type of denial
Beginning	The person can deny the thoughts and fantasy that come before the act. The person could deny planning or setting up the victim.
Middle	The person could deny specific acts he/she did. The person could deny the pain caused to the victim.
End	The person can deny bribes or threats that were made to the victim to keep the victim silent. The person can deny the harm caused to him/herself, to the victim, and to others.

Another problem that clients may encounter when completing this assignment is the desire to make the deviant sex act seem unimportant or unavoidable. In other words, a client may not deny the deviant sex act occurred but the client may not accept full responsibility for the act. Consider the ways that people could fail to accept responsibility for their behavior:

Minimize	Try to make something important appear small and insignificant.
Blame	Try to assign the responsibility for the act to someone else.
Justify	Try to make the act seem like it was okay and that it harmed no one.

Excuses   Try to explain that the act was
                 unavoidable and you could not
                 stop yourself.

Denial and responsibility are the two issues that
challenge the client when completing this assignment. It may be difficult to complete this assignment but clients who do complete it enter a new
world in which they can begin to feel positive
self-esteem.

Answer the following questions on a piece of
paper:

1. Recall a deviant sexual act that you committed.
   Who was the victim?
   When and where did the deviant sex occur?
   How old were you and the victim?
   How do you and the victim know each other?

2. Explain the reasons that you selected the
   victim.
   Was it a matter of convenience or were there
   other reasons?

3. How did you get the victim alone?
   Did you have to talk the victim into going
     somewhere with you?
   Did you just wait for everyone else to leave?
   How long had you planned the act?

4. What did you do to the victim?
   Where did you touch the victim?
   How did you touch the victim's body?
   Did you force the victim to touch your body?
   Describe all the things that you did to the
     victim?
   How long did the act last?

5. Describe what you said to the victim before,
   during, and after the act.

Describe what the victim said to you before,
during, and after the act.

6. Describe the resistance exhibited by the victim.
   Be sure to identify subtle resistance as well as
   obvious.

7. How did you feel immediately after the act?
   How did you feel the day after the act?
   How did you feel when the act was discovered?

8. How has your life changed as a result of this
   act?
   How has your action changed your family?
   What does your family think about this act?

STAGE ONE: CYCLE OF ABUSE
AND DEVIANT AROUSAL

Layout

My name is _____ .

My offense was _____ .

My victim was _____ .

My cycle of abuse includes _____
_____ .

I have had _____ cycle impulses since last group.

I controlled them by _____ .

My topic for today is _____
_____ .

Directions for Therapeutic Tasks

Positive and Deviant Sex Worksheet

Purpose: To educate clients about the criteria that separate positive sex from deviant sex.

Description: Most sex offenders have distorted ideas about sex. The purpose of this worksheet is to help the clients distinguish between positive sex and deviant sex. Positive sex promotes the spiritual, emotional, and physical health of both partners. Deviant sex does not.

Directions:

1. Read the Deviant and Positive worksheet in the Orientation section. Write a personal example for each of the criteria of deviant sex. Use

actual examples from your own sexual history to show you understand each characteristic. Write a personal example of the criteria of positive sex.

2. Present your examples in a group session. Accept feedback from group members.
3. Revise the worksheet as necessary.
4. Continue to use and refer to these criteria when discussing positive and deviant aspects of your own and peers' sexual behaviors and urges.

Offense Cycle Worksheet

Purpose: To help clients uncover and control their personal pattern of deviant sexual behavior.

Description: Each person has his/her own personal pattern of sexual behavior. Most people do not take time to uncover their own pattern of sex behavior. In the case of people who use deviant sex, it is important that they come to know their pattern of sexual behavior. It is only with self-awareness that a person can have self-control:

Self-Aware → Self-Monitor → Self-Control

The purpose of this worksheet is to help clients uncover their personal pattern of deviant sexual behavior. Once the pattern has been uncovered, clients will be expected to develop specific steps to interrupt the pattern and eliminate deviant sexual behavior.

In order to complete the offense cycle assignment, a client must know the steps of the offense cycle. The client must apply the steps to his/her life and discover his/her personal cycle of deviant sex.

A general description of the cycle is presented below:

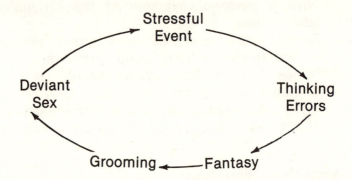

Stressful Event. A stressful event is any un-pleasant interaction or occurrences. Stressful events include things like an argument with a family member, physical abuse by a parent, a bad grade at school, or the death of a loved one.

Thinking Errors. People who use deviant sex have many thinking errors in their self-talk. The use of thinking errors creates negative self-talk.

Fantasy. A fantasy is the pictures in your mind. It is like a video of what you want to do. In the deviant sex cycle, fantasies are usually about how you will have sex with another person. Sometimes people masturbate while having a deviant sex fantasy.

Grooming. This is the time when the victim is set up. Grooming usually entails being nice to the victim so the victim will trust you. Grooming may also be such things as bribing, threatening, or lying to the victim.

Deviant Sex. This is the sex act that hurts the victim. Hurting the victim is a part of deviant sex. The person who uses deviant sex wants to have power over the victim. The victim is terrorized and humiliated by the other person's mixing of power and sex.

These five steps of the deviant sex cycle are present in everyone's pattern of deviant sexual behavior. How a person enacts each of the five steps is different depending upon the unique characteristics of that individual. The purpose of the therapeutic task described below is to help each client discover his/her personal deviant sex cycle.

Directions:

1. Get a pencil and paper. Answer the following questions. Notice that you will be working backward. That is, you will start by describing a deviant sexual act. Then you will describe how you groomed the victim. Then you complete the other steps in the cycle.
   a. *Deviant Sex*—Describe a deviant sex act. Indicate who, what, when, and where.
   b. *Grooming*—Describe how you set up the victim.
      How did you get the victim to trust you?
      What did you do to gain access to the victim?
      How did you keep your plan a secret?
      How did you isolate the victim or get the victim alone?
   c. *Fantasy*—Describe all the fantasies you had about sexual contact with the victim.
      What were the pictures in your mind?
      What did you want to do to the victim?
      How did you think the victim would react?
   d. *Negative Self-Talk*—

What thinking errors did you use regarding the stressful event?

What thinking errors did you use when you began to plan the deviant sex act?

e. *Stressful Event*—Give the date, time, and place of the stressful event that triggered the offense cycle.

2. Upon completing a draft of your Deviant Sex Cycle, orally present it to your group members during a group session.

3. Revise your Deviant Sex Cycle according to the feedback that you received.

4. Continue to revise and present the Deviant Sex Cycle until it is approved by your group members, your group therapists, and your primary therapist.

5. Complete an Offense Cycle worksheet for all your victims of deviant sex.

Covert Sensitization Worksheet

Purpose: To help clients decrease deviant arousal patterns while building positive alternatives.

Description: The first step in changing deviant arousal patterns is to increase self-awareness of these patterns. The preceding worksheets lead clients to recognize a deviant thought, but that is not enough. Clients must also learn to eliminate their deviant thoughts. This exercise leads a client to consider the negative consequences of acting on a deviant urge. Most offenders do not think through the deviant urge to consider the consequences of acting it out. It is hoped that by having the client think through to the end of an acting out, he will want to avoid it.

Covert sensitization is a three-step exercise. The

first step requires a client to describe a deviant urge or fantasy. The second step asks clients to write out *realistic* negative consequences. Most offenders say they were convinced they would never get caught. This step reminds them that it is possible to be caught and there are realistic negative consequences. Step three is a return to the positive. It is an opportunity for the clients to take an inventory of the good things in their life that they would lose if they acted deviant.

Directions:

1. Get some paper and a writing instrument.
2. On part one, write out the beginning of what could be a deviant sexual fantasy. Stop before any abuse occurs.
3. On part two, write out all of the negative consequences to you and others if you acted out this fantasy.
4. On part three, end by writing what positive things you could do instead that will have positive consequences for everyone.
5. Present this worksheet in a group session and revise it according to the feedback you receive.

Family Therapy

Purpose: To inform the client's family about therapeutic tasks addressed in stage one to increase accountability within the family.

Description: During stage one, the client must address three critical therapeutic issues: positive sexuality, offense cycle, and thinking errors. All three of these issues should be discussed in family therapy. The purpose of these discussions is quite simple: prepare the family system to accept the changes in the client when discussing positive sexuality; it is important for the family to take a look at itself. Values promoting healthy sex need to be clarified. The client and family need to openly discuss any behaviors or issues that have reinforced the client's deviant sexuality, such as premature exposure to adult sexual behaviors, lack of communication about healthy sex, and childhood access to sexually explicit media.

As the client recognizes the five steps of his/her personal offense cycle, the family can be educated by the client on what behaviors precede the deviant sex. As many families claim guilt and fear about not being able to trust the client, family members usually feel empowered to learn about the precursors of the abusive behavior. The client needs to be clear that breaking the cycle is his/her responsibility. The client needs to ask for help and accept help from the family when it holds him/her accountable for behaviors that could lead to offending.

The third issue the client can share in family therapy pertains to thinking errors. The client can discuss the thinking errors used most often to justify his/her behavior. The client can give examples of how these thinking errors support his/her offense cycle.

Directions:

1. The client can share the characteristics of healthy and deviant sex. The therapist can facilitate discussion among family members.
2. The client can use a large sheet of paper to graphically display the offense cycle while giving personal information about each step.
3. The client can bring his/her list of thinking errors to family therapy. The client explains the

thinking errors and gives examples of how he uses each one.

Positive Attitudes Group

Purpose: To teach the client how to recognize, control, and eliminate thinking errors and the exploitive behavior that results from thinking errors.

Description: The topic of thinking errors was first introduced to the client during orientation. While this presentation probably gave the client a working knowledge of thinking errors, the client has not been instructed to do anything more than recognize thinking errors. In the Positive Attitudes group, the client learns how to control and even eliminate thinking errors. The Positive Attitudes group is a closed-ended, short-term group that is four sessions in duration. The format of sessions is consistent: a thinking error is defined, clients are asked to identify examples of thinking errors in role-play scenarios, and homework assignments are given to self-monitor and correct thinking errors. The curriculum agenda for the Positive Attitudes group is listed below:

Session 1: Orientation
Session 2: Thinking Errors
Session 3: Thought Journal
Session 4: Control of Thinking Errors

The importance of controlling thinking errors cannot be overemphasized. Given the cognitive approach used in this Client Workbook, it should be readily recognized that much effort is devoted to changing the clients' thinking. It is assumed that thinking precedes all behavior. If thinking errors are eliminated then it is possible to reduce the behavior caused by thinking errors.

Directions:

1. Attend all scheduled sessions for the Positive Attitudes group.
2. While in group, use attending and listening skills.
3. When interacting with group members, be sure to give help and receive help.

STAGE TWO: VICTIM EMPATHY AND RESTITUTION

Layout

My name is _____ .

The person I hurt with deviant sexual behavior is

_____ .

I hurt this person by _____ .

In my lifetime, I have hurt _____ other people directly with my deviant sexual behavior.

Since my last group I have had _____ urges to hurt others using deviant sexual behavior.

My topic for today is _____ .

Directions for Therapeutic Tasks

Victim's Story

Purpose: To help the client see the deviant sexual act from the victim's point of view.

Description: When two people witness the same event, they each have different recollections of the event. This is true for just about any event. But when the event is an emotionally charged event, the difference in the way two people recall the event is extreme. Given the intense emotions of the perpetrator and the victim, it is certain that each would recall the episode differently.

There are other important differences in the ways in which the victim and perpetrator may recall the deviant sexual act. Perpetrators use thinking errors, and consequently the perpetrator will misread the situation and may even believe the deviant sexual act is desired. By contrast, the victim may be shocked that the perpetrator has introduced sexual behavior into the situation.

Another difference between the perpetrator and the victim would entail planning. The perpetrator plans the deviant sexual act and feels in control. On the other hand, victims are unaware of these plans and they feel confused and out of control when they get caught up in the perpetrator's plan.

There are many reasons why a victim and perpetrator see the deviant sexual act differently. The goal of this therapeutic exercise is to help clients recognize the differences and come to realize how shocked, confused, and controlled the victim felt during the deviant sexual act.

Directions:

1. Get some paper and a writing instrument. Write a script for one of your victims of deviant sex. The script is written from the victim's point of view, for example, "I felt him touch me."
2. Like any good script, there should be a beginning, middle, and end. Consider how the victim felt and thought at each point in the deviant sexual act. Try to capture the victim's feelings of shock and helplessness. Some of the issues you may wish to address may include:

   Beginning: The victim may believe he/she was minding his/her own business. The victim would not be able to read your mind and know your true intentions. The victim may have liked you and trusted you.

   Middle: The victim may be shocked as you begin to touch him/her in a sexual manner.

He/she may want you to stop but is too fearful to say so. The victim might experience physical pain. The victim probably has much confusion and many questions: Why me? What is going on here? How could he do this to me?

End: Did you threaten the victim? If so, how did that make the victim feel? Even if you did not threaten the victim, the victim feared future contact with you. Describe how the victim thought and felt after the deviant sexual act. Also, be aware that victims tend to blame themselves, for example, "What did I do to deserve this?" or "I must be a bad person because I was raped."

Once again, be sure to write the victim's story from the victim's point of view.

3. Present the victim's story during a group session and accept all feedback.
4. Continue to revise the victim's story until accepted by the group members and therapist.

"Forty Others" Worksheet

Purpose: To teach clients that impact of deviant sexual behavior is far-reaching and long-lasting.

Description: When the deviant sexual act concludes, the suffering is just beginning. Deviant sex would not be so painful if the suffering ended when the act ended. But that is not the case. Immediately after the deviant sexual act, the victim is consumed by confusion, sadness, and helplessness. Normal behavior and routines are interrupted. The intense feelings of shock and confusion may give way to prolonged sadness. Eventually the victim may begin to talk to family or friends about the incident, but not at first. The sexual victimization is never forgotten.

In discussing the deviant sexual act with others, the victim shares his/her pain. But there is a price that others must pay as they help the victim deal with this pain. Parents wonder what they could have done to prevent the act. They may even blame themselves for the act. Friends feel sad and helpless to aid the victim. Professionals who counsel or assist the victim recognize the needless waste and wonder, "What is society coming to?" A deviant sexual act does not just harm the person who is directly victimized. Everyone who comes in contact with the victim is victimized by the deviant sexual act.

To think that only those who come in contact with the victim are affected would be a narrow point of view. Actually, all of those who know the perpetrator are also victimized. The parents of the perpetrator may be shocked and blame themselves. Worse yet, the perpetrator's parents may get sued by the victim. The perpetrator's siblings may experience shame, loss of trust, or social isolation. And what about the professionals that deal with the perpetrator? These professionals must hear the account of the deviant sexual act and they must try to help the perpetrator prevent future acting out.

Overall, deviant sex affects many people. The effect is not short-term. Deviant sex causes pain for years even though the act may have lasted only minutes.

Directions:

1. Get some paper and a writing instrument.
2. Make a list of forty people who were harmed by one of your deviant sexual acts. Be sure to include the victim. Include any other person who was harmed by this behavior. Consider

people who already have been harmed by the behavior and those yet to be harmed. Indicate how each person was harmed.

3. Present your list in group. Accept feedback from group members and the group therapist. Revise the worksheet according to the feedback you receive.

4. Continue to present and revise the worksheet until it receives the approval of your group members and group therapist.

Clarification Letter

Purpose: To provide the victim(s) of deviant sexual act with the perpetrator's admission and explanation that the act was preplanned and totally the responsibility of the perpetrator.

Description: Victims require emotional restitution. Victims should learn directly from the perpetrator that no one is to blame for the deviant sexual act, except the perpetrator. So many times, victims claim some responsibility for their own victimization. They tell themselves that if they were only smarter, better, nicer, tougher, stronger, or quicker, none of this would have happened. For the victim, it can become all about them: What did they do to cause the perpetrator to act? What did they do wrong such that this was deserved? How did they contribute to being victimized? Did they fight or resist enough during the act?

All these questions would disappear if the perpetrator would just clarify what really went on during the deviant sexual act. Specifically, the perpetrator needs to clarify that the victim was set up and exploited and there was nothing that the victim did to cause or deserve this exploitation. It is through this clarification that victims learn an important lesson about being a victim: victims are not to blame for their own victimization. When the victim really learns this lesson, the victim can recapture some of the lost self-worth and self-esteem. Emotional restoration occurs.

One aspect of clarification needs discussion. Without a doubt, the perpetrator exerted power over the victim during the deviant sexual act. During clarification, the perpetrator is once again in a very powerful position. For example, the victim may know, and those around the victim may tell him/her, that he/she is not to blame for the deviant sexual act. Yet these words may have little impact upon the victim. However, when the victim comes face to face with the perpetrator and the perpetrator accepts complete responsibility for the act, the impact is liberating for the victim. Obviously, the perpetrator does have a special power that others do not have. The perpetrator has the power to set the record straight in a manner that no one else can. Special care needs to be taken to ensure that the perpetrator does not abuse this power as he/she did during the offense. That is why there are many restrictions placed upon the perpetrator during clarification. Conversely, the guidelines for clarification give the victim a great deal of control.

Directions:

1. The client must write a letter to his/her victim(s). The letter should adhere to the following format:
   a. *Greeting*: Write a script for what you will say to your victim at the beginning of the clarification session. You need to explain the purpose of the session. Tell the person

that you will be reading a letter. Explain the outline of the letter to the person. Let the person know that you will answer any questions. Ask permission to proceed.

b. *Selection*: Describe why you selected that person. Tell the person the good traits that he/she had that attracted you. Communicate how you used thinking errors to see the person as your victim.

c. *Setup*: Describe how you set up the person. Admit to the ways that you controlled the victim before the offense. Explain how you hid your true intentions while you did things to gain the person's trust. Describe all aspects of grooming.

d. *Description*: Describe the deviant sexual act in detail. Be sure that your description has a beginning, middle, and end. Be sure to include what you said and what the other person said during the beginning, middle, and end. Describe the ways that you continued to deceive and control the person throughout the offense. Describe what you did to control the person after the act. Describe how you tried to keep the deviant act a secret.

e. *Trauma Assessment*: Describe how the person resisted during the act. Explain that you knew the person was being harmed even at that time. Describe your understanding of how the person suffered since the time of the deviant sexual act. Identify all the other persons that your deviant sexual act has harmed.

f. *Conclusion*: Tell the person that the deviant sexual act was of your doing. Ask if it can be your responsibility to carry the burden of that act. Explain what you have done in treatment, what you have learned. Explain that it is your responsibility to change and stop using deviant sex. Encourage the person to feel safe from you.

2. After completing a draft of the letter, present it during a group therapy session. Accept all feedback. Revise the letter until you receive the approval of your group members and therapists.

Therapy Session with the Victim

Purpose: To provide the victim(s) with emotional restitution.

Description: A meeting between a victim and perpetrator is a strong emotional experience for all of those involved. It is, however, the emotional experience of the victim that is most critical. Victim–perpetrator meetings should occur only for the benefit of the victim. The goal of such meetings should be to provide a corrective emotional experience to the victim. This corrective emotional experience is often referred to as emotional restitution.

The positive effects of victim–perpetrator meetings often occur in surprising ways. For example, a victim may have a recollection of the perpetrator as an awesome bogeyman. Yet, when the victim and perpetrator meet, the victim immediately begins to realize that the perpetrator is not as big, mean, or smart as the victim's imagination had made the perpetrator. During the course of the clarification process, the perpetrator will have to self-disclose. By being vulnerable and self-disclosing, the perpetrator may enable the victim to recognize him/her as more human than superhuman. Overall, the effect of meeting with the perpetrator is to dispel many myths and misconceptions held by the victim.

One of the most problematic aspects of clarification is that the perpetrator still does have a special power with the victim that no one else has. The perpetrator has the power to know his/her intentions at the time of the deviant sexual act. Whereas other people can tell the victim that the perpetrator had planned the act and is totally to blame, when the perpetrator makes this statement it is powerful, more powerful than when anyone else says it. Therefore, much care needs to be exercised to ensure that the perpetrator does not re-victimize the victim during the meeting. That is why the perpetrator's comments to the victim have been carefully scripted in a letter.

The perpetrator should be required to adhere to the structure and contents of this letter. The perpetrator should speak only when spoken to. The victim should be allowed to determine when, where, and how the meeting is to occur. The victim should also be given the power to interrupt or stop the meeting. In general, tight control should be placed on the perpetrator and great control should be given to the victim in an effort to make sure that the power imbalance that started in the deviant sexual act does not continue.

Directions:

1. When the client has received approval from his/her group members and therapists, the

clarification letter is sent to the victim's therapist. The victim's therapist reviews the letter for accuracy and suggests modifications.

2. The client revises the letter according to the feedback of the victim's therapist. The letter is revised until approved by the victim's therapist.

3. A meeting between the victim and client is arranged. The victim is permitted to determine the time, date, and location of the meeting. The victim may have as many support persons available as desired. The perpetrator may have only his/her primary therapist present.

4. At the time of the clarification meeting, the victim, his/her supports and the therapists meet. The victim is told of the ways in which he/she controls the meeting. He/she can determine seating order, start time, and end time. The victim is told he/she has the power to interrupt or conclude the session at any time.

5. When the victim feels comfortable, the client is allowed to enter the room. The client is told where to sit. The client is told when to begin reading the clarification letter. The client can only read the letter or answer direct questions. The client cannot ask questions or make comments to others.

6. If the client tries to control the session or violates appropriate standards of conduct for this meeting, he/she will be ejected from the meeting.

7. After the client concludes reading the letter and answers all questions, he/she is dismissed. Those remaining may discuss the session.

8. Clarification may have to take place over several meetings.

9. Rather than a face-to-face meeting with the client, the victim is permitted to request an audiotape or videotape of the client reading the letter.

Sex Trauma Group

Purpose: To resolve issues pertaining to the client's experience as a victim of sexual abuse.

Description: Not everyone who commits a sex offense was sexually abused. Conversely, not everyone who is sexually abused goes on to become a perpetrator of deviant sex. Still, some persons who engage in deviant sex were themselves victims of sexual abuse. For these individuals it is important that they deal with the trauma of their abuse.

For those perpetrators who are victims of sexual abuse, the experience as a victim may motivate some deviant sexual acts. It is not uncommon for victims of sexual assault to develop confused and inappropriate notions about sexuality. For these confused individuals, it is no surprise when they engage in deviant sex. After all, they are so confused about sex, what else could they do?

Another common experience for perpetrators with a history of sexual abuse is that they attempt to relive the trauma so as to master it. Sex abuse is traumatic. The victim of sexual abuse suffers ongoing trauma after the abuse. In attempting to overcome the trauma, the abuse victim may wish to reenact the abuse, except that during the reenactment the person who was the victim tries to be the one in control. Since the only person in control in a deviant sexual act is the perpetrator, the person who was once a victim becomes a perpetrator.

There may be other reasons why a victim of sexual abuse might become a perpetrator. Regardless of the reason, one thing remains clear: two wrongs do not make a right. In other words, just because a person suffers sexual abuse it does not make it acceptable or excusable that he/she develops into a perpetrator. Remember, not everyone who is sexually abused becomes a perpetrator. Those perpetrators who were victims of sexual abuse must strive to understand how their abuse affected them and how it played a role in their behavior as a perpetrator. The bottom line is: perpetrators must recognize and control all aspects of their lives so as to prevent future sexual acting out.

Directions:

1. The client must enroll in the Sex Trauma group when his/her primary therapist indicates that the time is appropriate.
2. During Sex Trauma group sessions, the client adheres to group rules. The client makes special efforts to give help and receive help.
3. The client must complete all assignments required of Sex Trauma group participants.

Family Therapy

Purpose: To allow the client to share with family members work and progress that occurred during stage two.

Description: As was the case in stage one, in this stage there are issues that the client deals with during therapeutic activities that are also appropriate for discussion in family therapy. Some of the more noteworthy and important issues discussed in this stage of treatment that can also be discussed in family therapy include:

- Victim empathy
- The far-reaching impact of deviant sexual behavior
- The impact of the client's deviant sexual behavior on the client's family
- The client's experience as a sex abuse victim
- The experience of members of the client's family as sex abuse victims
- Exhibiting care and concern for family members
- Emotional restitution to family members

These are but a few of the more salient issues relevant for family therapy. Of course, other issues may be important depending upon the client's unique situation and the needs of family members.

Given that the theme of stage two is Victim Restitution, it would be appropriate for the client and his/her family members to explore how empathy, affection, and commitment are communicated in the family. Just as the client is learning to become more aware and responsive to the emotional needs of others, the client's family may need support for dealing with the same issue. In general, the family should take this time as an opportunity to strengthen their attachment to one another.

Directions:

1. The client's therapist attends a family session with the client. The therapist does not need to attend the entire session.
2. The client presents one of the Victim Restitution exercises to his/her family (e.g., "Forty

Others" worksheet). The client's therapist explains the purpose and rationale of the worksheet.

3. All those in the meeting discuss the worksheet presented by the client. Family members are encouraged to express feelings, thoughts, and experiences related to the worksheet.

STAGE THREE: RELAPSE PREVENTION AND POSITIVE AROUSAL

Layout

My name is _____ .

I am a person who made some bad choices and hurt _____ people by my deviant sexual behavior.

Since hurting these people I have learned techniques to control myself including _____
_____ .

Since the last group I have controlled _____ deviant urges.

My topic for today is _____ .

Directions for Therapeutic Tasks

ACE Worksheet

Purpose: To allow the client to develop specific coping skills for dealing with high-risk situations.

Description: The term *ACE* is an acronym for "Avoid – Cope – Escape." The three actions that are referenced in ACE are methods that the client can use to eliminate threats of relapse. Clients must learn that when they find themselves in a high-risk situation, they should "Play the ACE." That is, clients should avoid, cope with, or escape the situation.

Specific behaviors are required for each method of responding to high-risk situations. Consider the various ways a person could avoid, cope, or escape:

A. • Avoid people toward whom you have deviant urges.

- Avoid people who are deviant.
- Avoid places where you can gain access to victims.

C. • Use covert sensitization.
- Use a punishment scene.
- Use a rubber band.
- Recall Victim Restitution worksheets.

E. • Leave areas that promote deviant urges.
- Leave areas if potential victims are present.

The power of ACE is its simplicity. It is difficult to forget ACE once it is learned. ACE will always lead a person in the right direction, but the person must be willing to follow. It is important to understand that if a person does nothing in a high-risk situation, relapse is very likely. If a person plays the ACE, relapse is much less likely.

Merely knowing the ACE concept is not enough. A person must know when to use the ACE. The ACE should be used in all high-risk situations. There are basically two types of high-risk situations:

Temptations: Temptations come from the environment. People, places, or events can tempt a person to engage in deviant sex.

Urges: An urge comes from inside the person. Urges may take the form of sexual arousal but deviant urges usually contain the desire to dominate, control, or harm.

A high-risk situation is any situation in which the person has an urge or experiences temptation to engage in deviant sex. Temptations and urges can come at any time or place. That is why the person must always be ready to play the ACE.

Directions:

1. At least two ACE worksheets need to be completed and presented during a group therapy session. Each ACE worksheet should use the following format:

Temptation

A _____

    A _____

    C _____

    E _____

B _____

    A _____

    C _____

    E _____

Urge

A _____

    A _____

    C _____

    E _____

B _____

    A _____

    C _____

    E _____

The client should not be fooled by the illustration above. Actually, five urges and five temptations must be listed on each ACE worksheet.

2. The first ACE worksheet that the client completes should pertain to high-risk situations that could occur in the facility. The second ACE worksheet that the client prepares should pertain to participation in off-campus activities supervised by staff.

Other ACE worksheets should be prepared as dictated by the client's needs. For example, it would be important to develop an ACE worksheet for off-campus visits with family. It would also be useful to have an ACE worksheet completed for transitioning from residential care to community care. In general, the client should develop as many ACE worksheets as necessary to deal with threats of relapse.

High-Risk Situation Role Play

Purpose: To create a forum in which clients can practice and refine methods of dealing with high-risk situations.

Description: It is one thing to write down a method of dealing with high-risk situations but it is another thing to actually enact the coping response. Therefore, clients are given an opportunity to role play their ACE worksheets. The purpose of the role play is to help clients determine if their ACE worksheets are realistic. It would be rare if an ACE worksheet were totally unrealistic. Instead, it is expected that the role play will help the client modify and refine the ACE worksheet, thereby decreasing the likelihood of relapse.

It should be recognized that role play has been found to be very effective in teaching a variety of skills to many different types of persons with behavior problems. If the role play technique appears odd or unusual, clients should rest assured that role play can help in ways that paper and pencil worksheets never will be able to. Therefore, all those engaging in the role play should be encouraged about the possibility of learning new and better ways to prevent relapse.

Directions:

1. Using the ACE worksheet as a script, the client may prepare the role play. During the role play, the client will role play himself/herself. The client will try to enact the methods of dealing with high-risk situations. Other group members may role play persons referenced in the client's ACE worksheet. The therapist will help set up the role play. The client and others participating in the role play must have a clear idea of their roles. The script for the role play must have a beginning, middle, and end.
2. When everyone is sure about their roles, the role play may begin. A role play must be at least five (5) minutes in duration. More than one high-risk situation can be dealt with in the role play.
3. After the role play has concluded, the members of the role play discuss how it felt to be in the role play.
4. Everyone gives feedback to the client designed to help the client improve methods of dealing with high-risk situations.
5. The role play may be repeated based upon the feedback given to the client.

Relapse Prevention Plan

Purpose: To assist clients in developing coping strategies designed to prevent relapse, or a return to deviant or exploitive behavior.

Description: In the mid-1980s clinicians realized that it was easy to quit a negative or destructive behavior but it was difficult to stay quit. This problem began to be noticed in all kinds of treatment including treatment for eating disorders and chemical dependency, and in smoking cessation programs. So the issue of relapse began to receive a great deal of attention, and finally clinicians started to develop treatment programs aimed at overcoming problems with relapse. These treatment programs became known as relapse prevention programs.

Perhaps the single most important notion about relapse that must be understood is the notion that:

Relapse does not just happen.
Something always leads up to relapse.

Clients who have completed other therapeutic exercises in this workbook are familiar with the notion that there are warning signs that are obvious before a problem occurs. Those clients familiar with this notion also know the benefit of having early warning signs: If you recognize that a problem is about to occur, you can take steps to prevent the problem. That is what relapse prevention is all about—taking steps to prevent relapse.

From all that has been learned about relapse, a relapse process has been identified. The relapse process is displayed below:

Trigger → Seemingly Unimportant Decision → High Risk Situation → Lapse → Self-Doubt → Relapse

Trigger—This is any event, thought, or feeling that triggers the relapse process. It is usually a negative thought or feeling, or a conflict with an important person in your life.

Seemingly Unimportant Decision (SUD)—The SUD is a decision to put yourself in a high-risk situation or to talk yourself out of recognizing warning signs. For example, the child molester could convince himself that it is okay to volunteer at a school.

High-Risk Situation—A return to some mild form of deviant sexual behavior, for example, dissecting women, deviant masturbation, viewing pornography, any willful fantasizing about offending, or use of associated stimulation.

Lapse—This is a temporary setback. This is a place or action that makes a lapse possible by threatening one's self-control. This includes social pressure, negative emotional states, and interpersonal conflict, for example, a child molester being at a school in a room alone with a child. Being in a public place without wearing underwear is high risk for an exhibitionist.

Self-Doubt—Based upon the lapse the person looks at him/herself and becomes self-critical. The individual loses faith in him/herself. The individual doubts that he/she is capable of overcoming deviant sexual urges because the perceived gratification of relapse seems more powerful than pride of self-control.

Relapse—Due to the self-doubt and the satisfaction that the lapse created the person decides to engage in deviant sex.

As can be seen by the description of the relapse process, a relapse does not just occur. The person must take certain actions and make certain decisions for relapse to occur. Relapse is totally under the control of the individual. Consequently, relapse prevention plans can effectively interrupt relapse.

Directions:

1. Write a relapse prevention plan for your current situation. Get a piece of paper and list each step of the relapse process. Under each step of the relapse process leave space for five items. Your paper should look something like this:

Trigger

1

2

3

4

5

SUD

1

2

3

4

5

Be sure that you list *all* steps of the relapse process and leave five lines under each step.

2. For each of the five items, list a what-if. A what-if is a problem plus a solution. For example, under Trigger, you could write:

"What if I received a bad letter from home, I could let staff read it and discuss it with staff."

As can be seen by this format, every what-if

contains a problem and a solution. Since there are six steps in the relapse process, and five what-if's are needed for each step, your relapse prevention plan must contain thirty (30) what-if's.

3. Present your relapse prevention plan during a group therapy session. Accept the feedback that is offered. Revise the plan according to the feedback you receive. Continue to revise the plan until it is accepted by your group members and therapists.

Gender Issues Group

Purpose: To provide clients with information about human sexuality, sex roles, and sex stereotypes.

Description: When a person is growing up he/she is taught many things about human relationships. Of all the things that a person learns, perhaps the most important thing is how to relate to other people with dignity and respect. When a person can relate to others with dignity and respect, that person is capable of quality relationships.

Quality relationships are most important in intimate relationships. Sometimes what a person learns about intimate relationships actually interferes with the quality of the relationship. People who have learned negative or inappropriate ways of relating to others need to change. That is the purpose of the Gender Issues group: to help clients improve their ability to relate to others in a positive manner.

Some of the ingredients of a positive friendship have been discovered. Most researchers agree that the following elements are important to a quality friendship:

Loyalty—acting in a supportive manner; not causing harm to the other person.

Respect—accepting the person just as he/she is.

Enjoyment—feelings of satisfaction or happiness are derived from the relationship.

These qualities are typically present in any friendship relationship. These qualities should be present in same-sex and opposite-sex friendships.

Intimate relationships are very similar to friendship relationships. An intimate relationship has all of the same elements of a friendship plus two other important elements:

Exclusiveness—in an intimate relationship, a special bond is built between two people and they do not have that bond with anyone else.

Passion—the two persons desire physical contact with each other.

As can be seen, the intimate relationship is more complex than the friendship relationship because there are extra elements in an intimate relationship. However, neither type of relationship is easy to maintain. Friendships and intimate relationships require work. If you find that even with hard work it is difficult to maintain these types of relationships, then the Gender Issues group can probably be helpful.

Directions:

1. Attend the Gender Issues group as instructed by staff. Be on time for all meetings.
2. While in the Gender Issues group, be sure that you try to give help and receive help.
3. Do all assignments required by the staff who conduct the Gender Issues group.

Healthy Sexual Expression Worksheet

Purpose: To assist clients to develop positive sexual outlets for appropriate sexual desires.

Description: Positive sexual behavior occurs in the context of an exclusive relationship. The sexual contact between two persons in an exclusive relationship is meant to either support or strengthen the relationship. Each time sexual contact occurs between the two persons, both persons consent to the sexual contact. Both persons also consent to the type of sexual contact that occurs. There is no use of force, bribes, or trickery in positive sexual behavior.

It is important to understand that positive sexual expression occurs in the context of an exclusive relationship. This means that before sexual contact occurs between two people, the two people must first be friends. The friendship must be based upon respect, loyalty, and enjoyment of each other. Based upon the friendship, the two persons may become intimate. This means that the two persons make a commitment to each other and they feel sexual urges for each other. It is only after the two make their intimate relationship exclusive that sexual contact should occur.

In the context of an exclusive, intimate relationship, sexual behavior is actually a form of communication. Sexual behavior can communicate such things as "I love you" or "I trust you." When sexual behavior is used to communicate such messages, the sexual behavior can actually strengthen the relationship. At other times, sexual contact between two persons can communicate such things as "Let's play" or "You sexually arouse me." In such instances, the sexual behavior supports the relationship and reinforces the idea that the two people are committed and exclusive.

Even in an intimate relationship, there are times when one partner desires sexual contact but the other person is unwilling or unable. In this situation, sexual contact should not occur. Sexual behavior should occur only when both persons agree that the time is right to have sex. Just because two people have had sexual contact in the past does not mean that one of them can force the other to have sex at any time.

The type of sexual act that the couple engages in needs to be agreed upon by both persons. Sometimes one person wants to experiment with various sexual behaviors. Experimenting with sexual behaviors is natural and acceptable. It must be remembered, however, that even if one person wants to experiment, the other person must agree before the sexual act occurs. No threats, bribes, or manipulation should occur. No sexual contact should be harmful or degrading.

If one considers the various things that sexual contact can communicate, it should be recognized that there are several different types of appropriate sexual expression that can occur in an intimate, exclusive relationship:

> *Love*—expression of love and commitment
> *Play*—expression of mutual enjoyment
> *Experiment*—discovery of new sexual and intimate expressions

Positive sexual expression is exciting and powerful. When used correctly, positive sexual expression can make a relationship stronger and last longer.

Directions:

1. Write a script for positive sexual expression. Use the following outline:
   A. *Describe the Friendship* — How did you meet your intimate partner? What attracted you to him/her? Describe what you enjoy about your partner. What things do you have in common? Describe how each of you knows that you are loyal to each other. Describe how you know there is mutual respect for each other.
   B. *From Friendship to Intimacy* — Describe how you developed your exclusive relationship with your partner. How did you both agree to be exclusive? Describe how you began to communicate your sexual attraction to your partner. How did you maintain respect during this part of your relationship? How long did it take for you to become intimate?
   C. *Sexual Contact* — Describe how you and your partner agreed to have sexual contact. What did you say? What did your partner say? Describe your sexual contact with your partner. How did the sexual contact begin and end? What did you do during the sexual contact?
   D. *Positive Sexual Expression* — After your first sexual contact with your partner, describe how often you both have sexual contact. Describe the different types of sexual contact that you both have. Describe how the sexual contact supports or strengthens the relationship.
2. Upon completing the script for positive sexual expression, present it during a group therapy

session. Accept the feedback offered by group members and the therapists.

3. Continue to revise the script until it receives approval from your group members and therapists.

Family Therapy

Purpose: To provide a forum in which the client can share with family members all of the work attempted in stage three.

Description: In stage three, the focus is on relapse prevention and healthy sexual expression. These topics are certainly appropriate for discussion in family therapy. Moreover, it may be vital to the client's success that these topics are discussed during family therapy sessions.

For many clients, their original sexual acting out occurred at home. Obviously, there is a chance that relapse could occur in the home. Even for clients who have not sexually acted out at home, certain experiences in the home may either inhibit or contribute to relapse. Based upon these possibilities it is obvious that the client's relapse prevention work should be shared with the family in an attempt to help the family support the client's efforts to be successful.

Positive sexual expression should also be discussed during family therapy. The positive sexual expression discussed in this workbook is somewhat general. The client's family can help add detail to the client's notions of healthy sexual expression. Certainly, a discussion of healthy sexual expression can be powerful as it may give the client's parents an opportunity to repeat important messages and expectations about healthy sexual expression. Con sequently, the client may have the opportunity to include his/her family's expectations in his/her notions of healthy sexual expression.

Directions:

1. During a family therapy session, read one of your relapse prevention plans. Discuss the plan with your family members.
2. During a family therapy session, read one of your Positive Sexual Expression worksheets. Discuss the worksheet with family members. Accept feedback regarding your parents' expectations regarding healthy sexuality.

Assertiveness Skills Group

Purpose: To teach clients to meet their needs without harming or exploiting others.

Description: People who act out sexually sometimes feel so guilty that they become passive. They no longer try to meet their needs. They feel that if they try to meet their needs they will become aggressive or exploitive and harm someone. So rather than harm another person, or get in trouble for harming another person, they just do nothing. Their needs go unmet. They suffer but believe that the suffering is deserved or necessary. Unfortunately, such a person is very, very likely to relapse and engage in deviant sexual behavior.

Everybody has a right to meet his/her needs. People who do not meet their needs become frustrated and act out. It is not a matter of being either passive or exploitive. There is a middle ground. There is a way for a person to meet his/her needs without infringing on the rights of others. This way of behaving is called assertive.

When it comes to meeting needs, a person has three options:

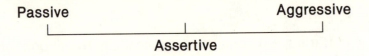

Passive — Do nothing; let others roll over you; do not meet your needs.

Assertive — Meet your needs without harming or exploiting others.

Aggressive — Meet your needs by use of threats, harm, or force; others are hurt.

Of the three ways to meet needs, only assertiveness is effective. If people are passive, they will not meet their needs. If people are aggressive, they may temporarily meet their needs but aggression usually causes more problems than it fixes. Thus, aggressive people will be swallowed up by the problems they create.

Assertiveness is effective because people can meet their needs and no one else is harmed. This means that problems are solved and no new problems are created. Assertiveness may be the most effective way of dealing with personal problems and personal needs.

Directions:

1. Attend the Assertiveness Training group as directed by the staff. Attend all group sessions. Complete all assignments. Give help and receive help while in group sessions.
2. Use new assertiveness skills in all aspects of your life.

STAGE FOUR: OUTPATIENT TREATMENT

Layout

My name is _____ .

I have made some important changes in the ways that I relate to others.

I am proud of the new ways I have learned to make friends and have intimate relationships.

This week I had _____ urges to do things the way I used to.
I coped with these urges by _____

_____ .

I would like to report the following program violations: _____

My topic for today is _____ .

Directions for Therapeutic Exercises

Schedule

Purpose: To allow the client to schedule his/her time in such a manner that relapse is less likely.

Description: There are two sayings that pertain to schedules:

1. Idle time is the devil's workshop.
2. People do not plan to fail. People just fail to plan.

With regard to the first saying, the point is rather obvious. When a person has unscheduled time, boredom may set in. In an attempt to overcome boredom, the person may engage in just about any activity. If the person has not properly thought about the activity, the activity may prove to be harmful. Recall the relapse process. Think about all the seemingly unimportant decisions and high-risk situations of the relapse process. If a person is not careful, these decisions and situations may creep up and unscheduled time may end up being the first step in the relapse process.

With regard to the second saying, the message is clear: you may not want to fail but if you do not make plans and stick to your plans, there is no way that you will succeed. Planning is the first step in accomplishing a goal. If a person fails to plan, the person will fail to reach the goal.

A schedule is a way to avoid both pitfalls of idle time and lack of plans. When a person develops a schedule, he/she is making use of the two most powerful personal resources: time and effort. A schedule gives direction to a person's time and effort. A schedule not only prevents problems associated with idle time, it also provides the person with the best possible chance to reach important goals.

Directions:

1. Get a piece of paper with lines on it. In the margin, list time in thirty-minute increments. Begin with the time 6:30 A.M. and list time until 10:00 P.M. Then, create seven columns on the paper and list the days of the week. Your paper should look like this:

	Sun	Mon	Tue	Wed	Thu	Fri	Sat
6:30–7:00							
7:00–7:30							
7:30–8:00							
8:00–8:30							
8:30–9:00							

and so on
to 10:00 P.M.

2. For every half-hour of every day of the week, list what you will be doing. Be sure to schedule school and work activities first.
3. When play or fun activities are listed, indicate what you will be doing and who will be participating in the activity along with you.
4. Present your daily schedule in a group therapy session. Receive feedback and modify your schedule according to the feedback that you receive.
5. The first daily schedule that you complete should pertain to your current situation. You should also develop a daily schedule for when you transition from this placement to home or your next placement.

Transition Plan

Purpose: To have the client prepare for transition from the current placement by making an explicit plan.

Description: As a person prepares to leave any place or group of people, two things typically occur. First, the person becomes nostalgic. *Nostalgic* is a term that means a person will look over the past and feel a mixture of happiness and sadness. Second, a person will feel nervous about going to a new place. This nervousness may be shown in many different ways, for example, increased energy, feeling worried, inability to sleep, and so on. When both nostalgia and nervousness occur together in a person, it is a strong emotional experience. Strong emotions can rob a person of his/her ability to cope. Therefore, it is important that people recognize and plan for nostalgia and nervousness when they go through a transition.

Planning for transitions can prevent a lot of trouble. Nostalgia and nervousness can make a person regress. When a person regresses, he/she falls back on old familiar patterns of behavior. When the person who regresses has a history of deviant sexual behavior, it is possible that a regression may increase the likelihood that the person will once again engage in deviant sexual behavior. If the person recognizes that a regression can cause a return to deviant sexual behavior, then he/she can make plans to avoid any activities that could result in sexual acting-out behavior.

In general, the value of a transition plan cannot be overestimated. A transition plan can help a person organize nostalgic thoughts and feelings. A transition plan can also help a person deal with his/her vagueness about making a change. Most importantly, a transition plan can help a person avoid regressed behavior and sexual acting out.

Directions:

1. Using the following outline, prepare your transition plan.
    A. *Nostalgia* — Describe what you were like when you entered the program. Describe how you have changed and what you are like now. What are the happiest, saddest, scariest, and angriest memories that you have about this treatment? Who helped you the most and had the biggest impact on you? How do you need to say good-bye to them? Write a general good-bye statement that applies to everyone else with whom you've come in contact.
    B. *Nervousness* — Describe the signs of nervousness you are aware of. What nervous thoughts are you having? How can you cope with your nervousness and nervous thoughts?
    C. *Regression* — Are you showing any signs of regression at this time? If so, what are they? What other signs of regression do you expect now? How will you be regressed after you leave this place? What do you need to do to cope?
    D. *What-if's* — Write twenty what-if's regarding the time after you leave this place. Your what-if's should pertain to adjusting to a new location and any regression that may occur.

2. Present your transition plan in a group therapy session. Accept feedback from your group members and therapists.
3. Revise your transition plan until it receives the approval of your group members and therapist.

REFERENCES

Abel, G. G., Becker, J. V., Cunningham-Rathner, J., et al. (1988). Multiple paraphilic diagnoses among sex offenders. *Bulletin of the American Academy of Psychiatry and Law* 16:153–168.

Abel, G. G., Becker, J. V., Mittleman, M., et al. (1987). Self-reported sex crimes of non-incarcerated paraphilics. *Journal of Interpersonal Violence* 2:3–25.

Adams, H. E., Motsinger, P. L., McAnulty, R. D., and Moore, A. L. (1992). Voluntary control of penile tumescence among homosexual and heterosexual males. *Archives of Sexual Behavior* 17:17–31.

Agee, V. L., and McWilliams, B. (1984). The role of group therapy in the therapeutic community in treating violent juvenile offenders. In *Violent Juvenile Offenders: An Anthology,* ed. R. A. Mathias, P. Demure, and R. S. Allison, pp. 283–296. San Francisco: National Council on Crime and Delinquency.

American Psychiatric Association. (1987). *Diagnostic and Statistical Manual of Mental Disorders,* 3rd ed. rev. Washington, DC: American Psychiatric Association.

Atcheson, J. D., and Williams, D. C. (1954). A study of juvenile sex offenders. *American Journal of Psychiatry* 3:366–370.

Bagley, C., and Schewchuk-Dunn, D. (1991). Characteristics of 60 children and adolescents who have a history of sexual assault against others: evidence from a controlled study. *Journal of Child and Youth Care,* Special Issue:43–52.

Bateman, A. J. (1948). Intra-sexual selection in *Drosophilia. Heredity* 2:349–368.

Baum, M. J. (1993). Neuroendocrinology of sexual behavior in the male. In *Behavioral Endocrinology,* ed. J. B. Becker, S. M. Breedlove, and S. Carter, pp. 97–130. Cambridge, MA: MIT Press.

Beach, F. A. (1976). Sexual attractively, preceptively and receptively in female mammals. *Hormones and Behavior* 7:105–138.

Becker, J. B., Breedlove, S. M., and Crews, D. (1993). *Behavioral Neuroendocrinology.* Cambridge, MA: MIT Press.

Becker, J. V., Kaplan, M. S., Cunningham-Rathner, J., and

Kavoussi, R. (1986). Characteristics of adolescent incest sexual perpetrators: preliminary findings. *Journal of Family Violence* 1:85–97.

Belmont, J. M., Butterfield, E. C., and Ferretti, R. P. (1982). To secure transfer of training. In *How and How Much Can Intelligence Be Increased?* ed. D. K. Detterman and R. J. Sternberg, pp. 147–154. Norwood, NJ: Ablex.

Bem, D. J. (1970). *Beliefs, Attitudes and Human Affairs.* Belmont, CA: Brooks/Cole.

Bengis, S. M. (1986). *A Comprehensive Service-Delivery System with a Continuum of Care for Adolescent Sexual Offenders.* Orwell, VT: Safer Society.

Berlin, F. S., and Meinecke, C. F. (1981). Treatment of sex offenders with antiandrogenic medication: conceptualizing, review and treatment modalities, and preliminary findings. *American Journal of Psychiatry* 138:601–607.

Blumer, D. (1970). Changes of sexual behavior related to temporal lobe disorders in man. *Journal of Sex Research* 6:173–180.

Breedlove, C. M. (1993). Sexual differentiation of brain and behavior. In *Behavioral Endocrinology,* ed. J. B. Becker, S. M. Breedlove, and D. Crews, pp. 39–70. Cambridge, MA: MIT Press.

Brinkman, A. S., McManus, M., Grapentine, W. L., and Alessi, N. (1984). Neuropsychological assessment of seriously delinquent adolescents. *Journal of the American Academy of Child Psychiatry* 23:453–457.

Carter, S. (1993). Neuroendocrinology of sexual behavior in females. In *Behavioral Endocrinology,* ed. J. B. Becker, S. M. Breedlove, and S. Carter. Cambridge, MA: MIT Press.

Cavanagh Johnson, T. (1988). Child perpetrators—children who molest other children: preliminary findings. *Child Abuse and Neglect* 12:219–229.

Coombs, R. H., and Kenkel, W. F. (1966). Sex differences in dating aspirations and satisfaction factors with computer-selected partners. *Journal of Marriage and the Family* 28:62–66.

Daly, M., and Wilson, M. (1983). *Sex, Evolution and Behavior,* 2nd ed. Belmont, CA: Wadsworth.

Davies, B. M., and Morganstern, F. S. (1960). A case of cysticercosis temporal lobe epilepsy and transvestism. *Journal of Neuro-*

logical and Neurosurgical Psychiatry 23:247–249.

Diamond, J. (1992). *The Third Chimpanzee: The Evolution and Future of the Human Animal.* New York: HarperCollins.

Ekman, P. (1985). *Telling Lies: Clues to Deceit in the Market Place, Politics and Marriage.* New York: W. W. Norton.

Famularo, R., Fenton, T., Kinscherff, R., et al. (1992). Differences in neuropsychological and academic achievement between adolescent delinquents and status offenders. *American Journal of Psychiatry* 9:1252–1257.

Fehrenbach, P. A., Smith, W., Monastersky, C., and Deisher, R. W. (1986). Adolescent sexual offenders: offender and offense characteristics. *American Journal of Orthopsychiatry* 56:225–233.

Ferrara, M. L. (1992). *Group Counseling for Juvenile Delinquents: The Limit and Lead Approach.* Newbury Park, CA: Sage.

———— (in press). *A Juvenile Sex Offender Treatment Program.* Laurel Lakes, MD: American Corrections Association.

Festinger, L. (1957). *A Theory of Cognitive Dissonance.* Evanston, IL: Row-Peterson.

Fields, H. S. (1978). Attitude toward rape: a comparative analysis of police, rapists, crisis counselors and citizens. *Journal of Personality and Social Psychology* 36:156–179.

Finkelhor, D., Araji, K. S., Baron, L., et al. (1986). *A Source Book on Child Sexual Abuse.* Newbury Park, CA: Sage.

Frisbie, L. V., Vanasek, F. J., and Dingman, H. F. (1967). The self and ideal self: methodological study of pedophiles. *Psychological Report* 20:599–706.

Gagne, P. (1981). Treatment of sex offenders with medroxyprogesterone acetate. *American Journal of Psychiatry* 138:644–646.

Galski, T., Thornton, K. E., and Shumsky, D. R. (1990). Brain dysfunction in sex offenders. *Journal of Offender Rehabilitation* 16:65–80.

Garrett, C. J. (1985). Effects of residential treatment on adjudicated delinquents: a meta-analysis. *Journal of Research in Crime and Delinquency* 22:287–308.

Gazzaniga, M. S., Steen, D., and Volpe, B. T. (1979). *Functional Neuroscience.* New York: Harper & Row.

Gebhart, P., Gagnon, J., Pomeroy, W., and Christianson, C. (1965). *Sex Offenders: An Analysis of Types.* New York: Harper

& Row.

Gendreau, P., and Ross, R. R. (1979). Effective correctional treatment: bibliotherapy for cynics. *Crime and Delinquency* 25:463–489.

_____ (1984). Correctional treatment: some recommendations for effective treatment. *Juvenile and Family Court Journal* 34:31–39.

_____ (1987). Revivification of rehabilitation: evidence from the 1980s. *Justice Quarterly* 4:349–408.

Gladue, B. A., Green, R., and Hellman, R. E. (1984). Neuroendocrine response to estrogen and sexual orientation. *Science* 225:1496–1499.

Goldberg, R. (1991). *Sit Down and Pay Attention: Coping with A.D.D. Throughout the Life Cycle.* Washington, DC: Psychiatric Institutes of America.

Goldstein, A. P. (1988). *The Prepare Curriculum: Teaching Prosocial Competencies.* Champaign, IL: Research Press.

Goldstein, K. (1952). The effects of brain damage on personality. *Psychiatry* 15:245–260.

Goldstein, M. J., Kant, H. S., and Hartman, J. J. (1973). *Pornography and Sexual Deviance.* Los Angeles: University of California Press.

Hammer, R. F., and Glueck, B. C. (1957). Psychodynamic patterns in sex offenders: a four factor theory. *Psychiatric Quarterly* 31:325–345.

Hart, S. D., Forth, A. E., and Hare, R. D. (1990). Performance of criminal psychopaths on selected neuropsychological tests. *Journal of Abnormal Psychology* 99:374–379.

Hendricks, S. E., Fitzpatrick, D. F., Hartmann, K., et al. (1988). Brain structure and function in sexual molester of children and adolescents. *Journal of Clinical Psychiatry* 49:108–112.

Howells, K. (1978). Some meanings of children for pedophiles. In *Love and Attraction,* ed. M. Cook and G. Wilson. London: Pergamon Press.

Hucker, S., Langevin, R., Dickey, R., et al. (1988). Cerebral damage and dysfunction in sexually aggressive men. *Annals of Sex Research* 1:33–47.

Izzo, R. L., and Ross, R. R. (1990). Meta-analysis of rehabilitation programs for juvenile delinquents: a brief report. *Criminal*

Justice and Behavior 17:134–142.

Kandel, E., and Freed, D. (1989). Frontal lobe dysfunction and antisocial behavior: a review. *Journal of Clinical Psychology* 45:404–413.

Kavoussi, R. J., Kaplan, M., and Becker, J. V. (1988). Psychiatric diagnosis in adolescent sex offenders. *Journal of American Academy of Child and Adolescent Psychiatry* 27:241–243.

Klüver, H., and Bucy, P. E. (1939). Preliminary analysis of functions of the temporal lobes in monkeys. *Archives of Neurology and Psychiatry* 42:979–1000.

Knopp, F. H. (1982). *Remedial Interventions for Adolescent Sex Offenses: Nine Program Descriptions.* Orwell, VT: Safer Society.

Knopp, F. H., Freeman-Longo, R., and Stevenson, W. F. (1992). *Nationwide Survey of Juvenile and Adult Sex Offender Treatment Programs and Models.* Brandon, VT: Safer Society.

Kolarsky, A., Freund, K., Machek, J., and Polak, O. (1967). Male sexual deviant: association with early temporal lobe damage. *Archives of General Psychiatry* 17:735–743.

Krgnicki, V. (1978). Cerebral dysfunction in repetitively assaultive adolescents. *Journal of Nervous and Mental Disease* 166:59–67.

Langevin, R. (1990). Sexual abnormalities and the brain. In *Handbook of Sexual Assault: Issues, Theories and Treatment of the Offender,* ed. W. L. Marshall, D. R. Laws, and H. E. Barbaree, pp. 103–113. New York: Plenum.

Langevin, R., Wortzman, G., Wright, P., and Handy, L. (1989). Studies of brain damage and dysfunction in sex offenders. *Annals of Sex Research* 2:163–179.

Lanyon, R. (1986). Theory and treatment of child molestation. *Journal of Consulting and Clinical Psychology* 54:176–182.

Lewis, D. O., Shankok, M. S., and Pincus, J. H. (1979). Juvenile male sexual assaulters. *American Journal of Psychiatry* 136:1194–1196.

Lipton, D. N., McDonel, E. C., and McFall, R. M. (1987). Heterosocial perceptions in rapists. *Journal of Consulting and Clinical Psychology* 55:17–21.

Maccoby, E. E., and Jacklin, C. N. (1974). *The Psychology of Sex Differences.* Palo Alto, CA: Stanford University Press.

Maclay, D. T. (1960). Boys who commit sexual misdemeanors. *British Medical Journal* 11:186–190.

Markey, O. B. (1950). A study of aggressive sex misbehavior in adolescents brought to juvenile court. *American Journal of Orthopsychiatry* 20:719–731.

McEwen, B. (1976). Interactions between hormones and nerve tissue. *Scientific American* 25:48–67.

Meloy, J. R. (1988). *The Psychopathic Mind: Origins, Dynamics and Treatment.* Northvale, NJ: Jason Aronson.

Meyer, W. J., Cole, C., and Emory, E. (1992). Depro Provera treatment for sex offending behavior: an outcome evaluation. *A Bulletin of the American Academy of Psychiatry and Law* 20:249–259.

Miller, B. L., Cummings, J. L., McIntyre, H., et al. (1986). Hypersexuality or altered sexual preference following brain injury. *Journal of Neurology, Neurosurgery and Psychiatry* 49:867–873.

Miller, L. (1992). The primitive personality and the organic personality: a neuropsychodynamic model for evaluation and treatment. *Psychoanalytic Psychology* 9:93–109.

Milloy, C. D. (1994). *A Comparative Study of Juvenile Sex Offenders and Nonsex Offenders.* Olympia, WA: Washington State Institute for Public Policy.

Mitchell, W., Falconer, M. A., and Hill, D. (1954). Epilepsy and fetishism relieved by temporal lobectomy. *Lancet* 2:626–630.

Moffit, T. E., Gabrielli, W. F., and Mednick, S. A. (1981). Socioeconomic status, IQ and delinquency. *Journal of Abnormal Psychology* 90:152–156.

Moffitt, T. E., and Silva, P. A. (1988). Neuropsychological deficits and self-reported delinquency in an unselected birth cohort. *Journal of American Academy of Child and Adolescent Psychiatry* 27:233–240.

Money, J. (1988). *Gay, Straight and In-between.* New York: Oxford University Press.

Murphy, W. D., Haynes, M. R., and Page, I. J. (1992). Adolescent sex offenders. In *The Sexual Abuse of Children: Clinical Issues,* vol. 2, ed. W. O'Donohue and J. M. Green, pp. 394–429. Hillsdale, NJ: Lawrence Erlbaum.

National Council of Juvenile and Family Court Judges. (1993). The revised report from the National Task Force on Juvenile Sex Offending. *Juvenile and Family Court Journal* 44:1–121.

Neidigh, L., and Krop, H. (1992). Cognitive distortions among child sexual offenders. *Journal of Sex Education and Therapy* 18:208–215.

Norman, D. K. (1976). *Memory and Attention: An Introduction to Human Information Processing.* New York: Wiley.

O'Brien, M. J. (1988). *Characteristics of male adolescent sibling incest offenders.* Orwell, VT: The Safer Society Program.

O'Connel, M. A., Leberg, E., and Donaldson, C. R. (1990). *Working with Sex Offenders: Guidelines for Therapist Selection.* Newbury Park, CA: Sage.

Overholser, J. C., and Beck, S. (1986). Multi-method assessment of rapists, child molesters, and three control groups on behavioral and psychological measures. *Journal of Consulting and Clinical Psychology* 54:683–687.

Parmely, M. (1994). *A Single-Subject Time Serves Investigation of Script Theory in Aphasia Intervention.* Thesis, Texas Technical University.

Pithers, W. D., Cumming, G., Beal, L., et al. (1988). Relapse prevention. In *Appropriation Guide to Treating the Incarcerated Male Sex Offender,* ed. B. K. Schwartz and H. R. Cellini, pp. 123–140. Washington, DC: National Institute of Corrections.

Pontius, A. A. (1974). Basis for a neurological test of frontal lobe system functioning up to adolescence. *Adolescence* 9:221–232.

Pontius, A. A., and Ruttiger, K. I. (1976). Frontal lobe system maturational lag in juvenile delinquents shown in narrative tests. *Adolescence* 11:509–518.

Robbins, M. (1989). Primitive personality organization as an interpersonally adaptive modification to cognition and effect. *International Journal of Psychoanalysis* 70:443–459.

Ryan, G. D., and Lane, S. L. (1991). *Juvenile Sexual Offending: Causes, Consequences and Correction.* Lexington, MA: Lexington.

Sade, D. S. (1968). Inhibition of son–mother mating among free ranging rhesus monkeys. *Science and Psychoanalysis* 12:18–37.

Saunders, E., Awad, G. A., and White, G. (1986). Male adolescent sexual offenders: the offender and the offense. *Canadian Journal of Psychiatry* 31:542–548.

Schuell, H., Jenkins, J., and Jimenez-Pabon, E. (1964). *Aphasia in Adults.* New York: Harper & Row.

Schuster, R., and Guggenheim, P. D. (1982). An investigation of intellectual capabilities of juvenile delinquents. *Journal of Forensic Science* 27:393–400.

Segal, Z. V., and Marshall, W. L. (1985). Heterosexual social skills of rapists and child molesters. *Journal of Consulting and Clinical Psychology* 53:55–63.

Segal, Z. V., and Stermac, L. E. (1984). A measure of rapists' attitudes toward women. *International Journal of Law and Psychiatry* 7:219–222.

_____ (1990). The role of cognition in sexual assault. In *Handbook of Sexual Assault: Issues, Theories and Treatment of the Offender,* ed. W. L. Marshall, D. R. Laws, and H. E. Barbaree. New York: Plenum.

Shoor, M., Speed, M. H., and Bartest, C. (1966). Syndrome of the adolescent child molester. *American Journal of Psychiatry* 122:783–789.

Spellacy, F. (1977). Neurological differences between violent and nonviolent adolescents. *Journal of Clinical Psychology* 33:966–969.

Stevens, J., Sachder, K., and Melstein, V. (1968). Childhood and the electroencephalogram. *Archives of Neurology* 17:160–177.

Swabb, D. F., and Fliers, E. (1985). A sexually dimorphic nucleus in the brain. *Science* 228:1112–1115.

Tarter, R. E., Hegedus, A. M., Allerman, A. I., and Katz-Garcis, L. (1983). Cognitive capacities of juvenile, violent, nonviolent and sexual offenders. *Journal of Nervous and Mental Disease* 171:564–567.

Thornhill, R. (1976). Sexual selection and feeding behavior in Bittacus appicals. *American Naturalist* 110:529–548.

Toglia, J. P. (1991). Generalization of treatment: a multicontext approach to cognitive perceptual impairment in adults with brain injuries. *American Journal of Occupational Therapy* 45:505–516.

Tompkins, C. A. (1991). Redundancy enhances emotional inferencing by right and left hemisphere damaged adults. *Journal of Speech and Hearing Research* 34:1142–1149.

Tsushima, W. T., and Wedding, D. (1979). A comparison of the Halstead-Reitan neurological battery and computerized topography in the identification of brain dysfunction. *Journal of Nervous and Mental Disease* 167:704–707.

Turner, C. H. (1981). *Maps of the Mind*. New York: Macmillan.

Utamsing, M. C. L., and Holloway, R. L. (1982). Sexual dimorphism in the human corpus callosum. *Science* 216:1431–1432.

Yeudall, L. T., Fromm-Auch, D., and Davies, P. (1982). Neuropsychological impairment of persistent delinquency. *Journal of Nervous and Mental Diseases* 170:257–265.

Yochelson, S., and Samenow, S. (1976). *The Criminal Personality,* vols. 1 and 2. New York: Jason Aronson.

Wade, J. A., Clark, R., and Hamm, A. (1975). Cerebral hemispheric asymmetry in humans. *Archives of Neurology* 32:239–246.

Wolfgang, M. E., Figlio, R. M., and Sellin, T. (1972). *Delinquency in a Birth Cohort*. Chicago: University of Chicago Press.

INDEX

About the Authors

Matthew Ferrara, Ph.D., works exclusively with forensic clients in private practice in Austin, Texas. He has developed specialized sex offender treatment programs for high risk offenders, incest perpetrators, developmentally delayed offenders, and offenders in denial. Formerly, as chief of counseling for the Texas Youth Commission, Dr. Ferrara designed and implemented the agency's group therapy program and substance abuse treatment services. He was also the chief psychologist for the Texas prison system, where he was responsible for all mental health policy and services and created the agency's 200-bed sex offender treatment program. Dr. Ferrara's current work with neurologically impaired sex offenders represents a continuing effort to render specialized treatment to high-risk populations.

Sherry Gaffin McDonald, L.M.S.W.-A.C.P., lectures nationally in the field of clinical social work with adolescents. She is a full-time clinician specializing in the treatment of adolescents with sexual disorders, sexual paraphilias, juvenile sexual offenders, and adolescent victims of sexual abuse. She is currently the lead therapist for the Sexual Treatment Services Department at the San Marcos Treatment Center in San Marcos, Texas.